I0888439

Revolutionizing Medicine With Autonomous Robotics

Dattatray Gopal Takale
https://orcid.org/0000-0002-8241-3989
Vishwakarma Institute of Information Technology, India

Parikshit N. Mahalle
https://orcid.org/0000-0001-5474-6826
Vishwakarma Institute of Information Technology, India

Bipin Sule
Vishwakarma Institute of Technology, India

Vivek S. Deshpande
Vishwakarma Institute of Information Technology, India

Nilesh P. Sable
https://orcid.org/0000-0002-5855-4087
Vishwakarma Institute of Information Technology, India

IGI Global
Scientific Publishing
Publishing Tomorrow's Research Today

Vice President of Editorial Melissa Wagner
Director of Acquisitions Mikaela Felty
Director of Book Development Jocelynn Hessler
Production Manager Mike Brehm
Cover Design Jose Rosado

Published in the United States of America by
IGI Global Scientific Publishing
701 East Chocolate Avenue
Hershey, PA, 17033, USA
Tel: 717-533-8845 | Fax: 717-533-7115
Website: https://www.igi-global.com E-mail: cust@igi-global.com

Copyright © 2026 by IGI Global Scientific Publishing. All rights reserved. No part of this publication may be reproduced, stored or distributed in any form or by any means, electronic or mechanical, including photocopying, without written permission from the publisher. Use of this publication to train generative artificial intelligence (AI) technologies is expressly prohibited. The publisher reserves all rights to license its use for generative AI training and machine learning model development.

Product or company names used in this set are for identification purposes only. Inclusion of the names of the products or companies does not indicate a claim of ownership by IGI Global Scientific Publishing of the trademark or registered trademark.

Library of Congress Cataloging-in-Publication Data

(CIP Data Pending)
ISBN13: 9798337301792
Isbn13Softcover: 9798337301808
EISBN13: 9798337301815
British Cataloguing in Publication Data
A Cataloguing in Publication record for this book is available from the British Library.

All work contributed to this book is new, previously-unpublished material.
The views expressed in this book are those of the authors, but not necessarily of the publisher.
This book contains information sourced from authentic and highly regarded references, with reasonable efforts made to ensure the reliability of the data and information presented. The authors, editors, and publisher believe the information in this book to be accurate and true as of the date of publication. Every effort has been made to trace and credit the copyright holders of all materials included. However, the authors, editors, and publisher cannot assume responsibility for the validity of all materials or the consequences of their use. Should any copyright material be found unacknowledged, please inform the publisher so that corrections may be made in future reprints.

To our family, for their endless love, patience, and encouragement; and to all the dedicated professionals, researchers, and students striving to transform healthcare through innovation in robotics and artificial intelligence.

Your passion and commitment make this work meaningful.

Table of Contents

Detailed Table of Contents

when compared to normal tissues. Thus, the utilization of CNNs for classifying and detecting brain tumors is quite efficient, provided the combined application of the CLAHE algorithm to boost the image contrast, where the outcomes of the classification attained a high accuracy. This chapter reflects on the Sustainable Development Goals in general by contributing to the development of more effective diagnostic tools and, consequently, enhancing the health of individuals. It is in line with the need to have sustainable healthcare systems for the constant and fair diagnosis and treatment of brain tumors regardless of the climate situation.

Chronic diseases, including diabetes, cardiovascular disorders, and cancer, are responsible for more than 70% of deaths worldwide, placing considerable pressure on healthcare systems. This chapter explores the revolutionary impact of artificial intelligence in the management of chronic illnesses. By utilizing machine learning, AI can predict disease progression and offer highly accurate personalized treatment options. It enhances diagnostic processes, supports remote patient monitoring through wearable technology, and allows for real-time management of treatments, thereby improving patient outcomes. Significant topics covered include AI applications for the early detection of diabetic retinopathy and cancer, customized treatment plans, and automated medication management. Additionally, AI improves telemedicine by facilitating at-home monitoring of chronic conditions through the collection of real-time data. The chapter also addresses challenges such as data privacy and biases in AI, highlighting the importance of ethical considerations.

The global healthcare problem of chronic kidney disease (CKD) requires accurate predictions in the early stages to achieve appropriate treatment and management strategies. Deep learning through deep neural networks (DNNs) has received rising interest for CKD prediction systems because it effectively combines medical images with clinical information. The review investigates the implementation of

Embryo selection plays a critical role in the success of In Vitro Fertilization (IVF), yet conventional methods relying on morphological assessment and expert judgment are often subjective and inconsistent. To address these limitations, this study investigates the application of machine learning (ML) algorithms for automated, objective, and accurate embryo classification. A comparative analysis was conducted on six prominent ML models: Support Vector Machine (SVM), Random Forest (RF), k-Nearest Neighbors (k-NN), Convolutional Neural Network (CNN), ResNet, and ConvNeXT. Publicly available datasets, including IVF time-lapse sequences and the Early Embryo Viability Assessment (Eeva) dataset, were utilized for training and validation. Evaluation metrics such as accuracy, precision, recall, F1-score, and Area Under the Curve (AUC) were employed to assess model performance. The results show that deep learning models, especially ConvNeXT and ResNet, performed better than traditional algorithms, reaching accuracy scores over 93% and high AUC values.

Chronic Kidney Disease (CKD) is a progressive and often asymptomatic condition that poses significant health risks if not detected early. With recent advances in machine learning (ML), predictive models have been developed to enable early CKD diagnosis using clinical data. This study presents a comparative review of existing ML-based approaches applied to datasets such as the UCI CKD dataset and electronic health records (EHRs). It examines algorithms like Logistic Regression, Support Vector Machine (SVM), Random Forest, K-Nearest Neighbors (KNN), and XGBoost. The models are compared using metrics such as accuracy, precision,

Foreword

Healthcare is undergoing a profound transformation driven by unprecedented advances in artificial intelligence, autonomous robotics, and data-driven technologies. The integration of these intelligent systems into medical environments is not merely an enhancement of existing practices it represents a fundamental shift in how clinicians diagnose, monitor, and treat patients. As we transition toward precision medicine, smart hospitals, and automated care systems, the need for comprehensive scholarship capturing this evolution has never been greater.

Revolutionizing Medicine with Autonomous Robotics arrives at a pivotal moment in this technological renaissance. This edited volume brings together leading researchers, practitioners, and innovators who expertly articulate the opportunities, challenges, and real-world applications of autonomous systems in modern healthcare. The chapters cover a remarkable range of topics, from surgical robotics and AI-assisted diagnostics to intelligent patient monitoring, telemedicine automation, and next-generation rehabilitation and caregiving solutions. Each contribution reflects rigorous scientific inquiry, practical relevance, and a forward-looking perspective that is essential for understanding the future trajectory of medical technology.

The strength of this book lies not only in its breadth of topics but also in its interdisciplinary nature. Robotics engineers, clinicians, AI scientists, biomedical researchers, and policy analysts offer complementary viewpoints that emphasize the collaborative spirit needed to responsibly advance autonomous healthcare. Their insights underscore critical issues related to ethics, data privacy, algorithmic fairness, regulatory frameworks, and patient trust—factors that will shape the successful adoption of autonomous systems in real-world clinical settings.

By presenting both foundational knowledge and cutting-edge innovations, this book serves as an invaluable resource for academicians, healthcare professionals, students, policymakers, and industry leaders. It equips readers with a nuanced understanding of how intelligent automation can enhance accuracy, reduce clinical workload, improve patient outcomes, and drive a more efficient healthcare ecosystem. Simultaneously, it encourages thoughtful consideration of the societal implications, ensuring that progress is guided by responsibility, transparency, and human-centered values.

As the global healthcare landscape evolves, autonomous robotics and AI will continue to redefine what is possible in medicine. This volume not only documents that transformation but also inspires new directions for research, development, and implementation. It is a significant and timely contribution to the scholarly dialogue and a testament to the dedication of the editors and contributing authors who have thoughtfully curated this work.

It is with great pleasure that I commend *Revolutionizing Medicine with Autonomous Robotics* to readers worldwide. May it spark innovation, inform practice, and guide the future of intelligent healthcare systems.

Preface

The convergence of artificial intelligence (AI), autonomous robotics, and advanced data-driven technologies is transforming healthcare at an unprecedented pace. What once belonged in the realm of science fiction robots assisting surgeons, intelligent systems predicting patient deterioration, autonomous monitoring devices assessing vital signs, or AI tools identifying diseases before symptoms appear has now become a tangible reality. This book, *Revolutionizing Medicine with Autonomous Robotics*, brings together these groundbreaking advancements to present a comprehensive, forward-looking view of how autonomous systems are reshaping modern medical practice.

Healthcare today stands at a crucial inflection point. The rising burden of chronic diseases, aging populations, growing demand for precision medicine, and the need for cost-effective solutions have created an environment where traditional methods are no longer sufficient. Autonomous systems, powered by AI, machine learning, robotics, big data, and IoT-driven connectivity, offer transformative solutions that promise greater accuracy, efficiency, safety, and personalization. The motivation for this book arises from this global shift an urgent need to understand, evaluate, and adopt next-generation technologies that can improve clinical outcomes, reduce human error, and expand access to quality healthcare.

The accepted chapters in this book collectively provide a comprehensive exploration of how autonomous robotics and artificial intelligence are transforming modern healthcare. The opening chapters establish the technological foundation by introducing essential concepts of AI, robotics, machine learning, IoT, and healthcare data management, along with critical discussions on ethics, security, and regulatory frameworks. Subsequent chapters examine the rapidly evolving field of surgical robotics, highlighting robotic-assisted interventions, precision enhancement, and autonomous capabilities now entering the operating room. The book then transitions into AI-driven diagnostics, presenting breakthroughs in radiology, pathology, genomics, and early disease detection through advanced analytical models and smart diagnostic devices. Further chapters focus on autonomous patient-care systems—

including AI-enabled patient monitoring, rehabilitation robots, telemedicine automation, chronic disease management technologies, and supportive systems for elderly care—demonstrating how intelligent tools improve safety, personalization, and continuity of care. The final set of chapters offers future-oriented insights into technological trends, implementation challenges, interdisciplinary collaboration, and workforce development, outlining a clear roadmap for integrating autonomous systems into global healthcare practice.

ORGANIZATION OF THE BOOK

Chapter 1: Impact of NAMI Robots on Collision Detection, Avoidance, and Applications

This chapter includes the implementation, applications, benefits, and potential of Navigational Autonomous Mapping Interface (NAMI) robots. NAMI robots, designed with advanced sensing, perception, and decision-making capabilities, utilize a combination of sensors, machine learning algorithms, and real-time data processing to improve their interaction with dynamic environments. It has a considerable impact on collision detection and collision avoidance into industrial application. The NAMI robot is a humanoid designed with multiple advances sensors and able to takes decision based on received sensor values to avoid collision. NAMI robots can explore unknown territories without causing damage to them. It proves to be a valuable tool for exploration and information support.

Chapter 2: AI in Patient Monitoring

The chapter underscores the significance of enhanced decision support tools which helps medical professionals to make more informed and quicker and better clinical judgements, ultimately improving patient care. It also highlights the potential for AI to reduce healthcare costs through early detection of health issues and prevention of complications, leading to fewer hospital readmissions and more efficient use of healthcare resources. The chapter also touches on the importance of building patient trust and acceptance of AI technologies through transparent communication about their benefits, limitations, and ethical use. By addressing these critical aspects, the chapter provides a comprehensive overview of how AI is poised to revolutionize medicine, improving patient outcomes, enhancing healthcare delivery, and shaping the future of medical practice.

Chapter 3: A Review of Pre-Pregnancy Health Risk Assessment in Women Current Practices and Emerging Trends

Pre-pregnancy health assessment is crucial for identifying and managing risk factors affecting maternal and fetal health. This paper reviews traditional approaches like routine medical exams, lifestyle evaluations, and basic health metrics, noting their limitations in precision and personalization, especially for diverse populations. To bridge these gaps, the paper explores advanced methods such as artificial intelligence (AI), soft computing, genetic profiling, and wearable technologies. AI-driven models and techniques like fuzzy logic show potential in improving predictive accuracy, while wearable devices enable real-time health monitoring for proactive care. The paper underscores the need for a holistic, personalized risk assessment framework integrating various health metrics, advocating for interdisciplinary collaboration to enhance outcomes in maternal and infant health, and providing a foundation for researchers and clinicians to advance pre-pregnancy care.

Chapter 4: Revolutionizing Brain Tumor Detection by Exploring the Environmental Impact and Deep Learning in MRI Segmentation

Maligancy of the brain is a disorder that affects the health of populations worldwide and for diagnosis, calls for complex skills and high-resolution techniques. This work proposes the use of a new strategy for the detection and segmentation of brain tumors with the help of MRI images. Concerning MRI, although the tumors are high in water content and possess hydrogen atoms, they give variations in signal intensity when compared to normal tissues. Thus, the utilization of CNNs for classifying and detecting brain tumors is quite efficient, provided the combined application of the CLAHE algorithm to boost the image contrast, where the outcomes of the classification attained a high accuracy. This chapter reflects on the Sustainable Development Goals in general by contributing to the development of more effective diagnostic tools and, consequently, enhancing the health of individuals. It is in line with the need to have sustainable healthcare systems for the constant and fair diagnosis and treatment of brain tumors regardless of the climate situation.

Chapter 5: AI in Managing Chronic Diseases: AI in Managing Chronic Diseases

Chronic diseases, including diabetes, cardiovascular disorders, and cancer, are responsible for more than 70% of deaths worldwide, placing considerable pressure on healthcare systems. This chapter explores the revolutionary impact of artificial intelligence in the management of chronic illnesses. By utilizing machine learning, AI can predict disease progression and offer highly accurate personalized treatment options. It enhances diagnostic processes, supports remote patient monitoring through wearable technology, and allows for real-time management of treatments, thereby improving patient outcomes. Significant topics covered include AI applications for the early detection of diabetic retinopathy and cancer, customized treatment plans, and automated medication management. Additionally, AI improves telemedicine by facilitating at-home monitoring of chronic conditions through the collection of real-time data. The chapter also addresses challenges such as data privacy and biases in AI, highlighting the importance of ethical considerations.

Chapter 6: Systematic Review of Medical Imaging and Clinical Data in CKD Prediction Using Deep Neural Networks

The global healthcare problem of chronic kidney disease (CKD) requires accurate predictions in the early stages to achieve appropriate treatment and management strategies. Deep learning through deep neural networks (DNNs) has received rising interest for CKD prediction systems because it effectively combines medical images with clinical information. The review investigates the implementation of deep neural networks for predicting CKD by uniting medical imaging approaches with clinical database information. Medical imaging techniques using ultrasound as well as CT scans and MRI, together with clinical datasets, generate important information regarding the initial development stages of CKD. The enormous computing ability of DNNs makes them perfect for detecting intricate patterns that standard evaluation techniques typically overlook. The article investigates multiple DNN structures predicting CKD, system performance levels, obstacles, and possible future enhancements.

Chapter 7: Evaluating VGG16, ResNet50, and Xception for COVID-19 Detection via a Web-Based Deep Learning Interface

The global outbreak of COVID-19 has emphasized the need for fast and accurate diagnostic methods, especially in areas where advanced testing facilities are scarce or unavailable. This research proposes a deep learning-based method for the binary classification of chest X-ray images aimed at detecting COVID-19 infections. We evaluate and compare the performance of three prominent Convolutional Neural Network (CNN) architectures ResNet50, VGG16, and Xception trained on publicly available chest radiograph datasets. Additionally, a confusion matrix, training versus validation accuracy plots, and the ROC curve are employed to gain deeper insights into the model's effectiveness and diagnostic capability. To enhance usability, a user-friendly web interface has also been developed, enabling users to upload images and obtain real-time classification results. Experimental findings indicate that all three models perform well in distinguishing COVID-19 cases, with the Xception model achieving the highest accuracy.

Chapter 8: A Comparative Study of Machine Learning Algorithms for Embryo Selection in In Vitro Fertilization

Embryo selection plays a critical role in the success of In Vitro Fertilization (IVF), yet conventional methods relying on morphological assessment and expert judgment are often subjective and inconsistent. To address these limitations, this study investigates the application of machine learning (ML) algorithms for automated, objective, and accurate embryo classification. A comparative analysis was conducted on six prominent ML models: Support Vector Machine (SVM), Random Forest (RF), k-Nearest Neighbors (k-NN), Convolutional Neural Network (CNN), ResNet, and ConvNeXT. Publicly available datasets, including IVF time-lapse sequences and the Early Embryo Viability Assessment (Eeva) dataset, were utilized for training and validation. Evaluation metrics such as accuracy, precision, recall, F1-score, and Area Under the Curve (AUC) were employed to assess model performance. The results show that deep learning models, especially ConvNeXT and ResNet, performed better than traditional algorithms, reaching accuracy scores over 93% and high AUC values.

Chapter 9: Machine Learning-Based Comparative Analysis for Chronic Kidney Disease Prediction Using Clinical Data

Chronic Kidney Disease (CKD) is a progressive and often asymptomatic condition that poses significant health risks if not detected early. With recent advances in machine learning (ML), predictive models have been developed to enable early CKD diagnosis using clinical data. This study presents a comparative review of existing ML-based approaches applied to datasets such as the UCI CKD dataset and electronic health records (EHRs). It examines algorithms like Logistic Regression, Support Vector Machine (SVM), Random Forest, K-Nearest Neighbors (KNN), and XGBoost. The models are compared using metrics such as accuracy, precision, recall, F1-score, and AUC-ROC. Results from reviewed studies show that ensemble methods, particularly Random Forest and XGBoost, offer superior performance and robustness in managing missing or imbalanced data. Additionally, the study highlights variations in data preprocessing, feature selection, and validation strategies.

What sets this book apart is its comprehensive and interdisciplinary approach. Scholars, clinicians, engineers, technologists, and industry leaders have collaborated to create a unified, authoritative resource that bridges technical innovation with clinical application. This diversity ensures that each chapter provides both scientific depth and real-world relevance.

The insights presented in this book will benefit a wide audience—researchers aiming to push the boundaries of AI-driven healthcare, practitioners adopting robotics and automation in clinical workflows, policymakers designing future regulations, educators updating curricula, and industry innovators developing next-generation medical technologies. The global list of contributing authors demonstrates the collaborative spirit required to advance the field and reflects perspectives from medicine, engineering, computer science, law, policy, and industry.

As AI and autonomous robotics continue to redefine medicine, it is essential for stakeholders across the healthcare ecosystem to understand not only what these technologies can achieve, but also how to deploy them responsibly, ethically, and sustainably. We hope that *Revolutionizing Medicine with Autonomous Robotics* serves as an inspiring and practical guide one that empowers readers to contribute to this transformative journey and to shape the future of medical care.

It is our belief that the knowledge, research, and vision encapsulated in this book will catalyze innovation, fuel interdisciplinary collaboration, and support the next generation of breakthroughs in intelligent healthcare systems. As autonomous robotics and AI move from innovation to integration, this book stands as both a roadmap and a reflection of the remarkable evolution occurring at the intersection of medicine, technology, and human progress.

Acknowledgement

The editors of *Revolutionizing Medicine with Autonomous Robotics* extend their sincere appreciation to all contributing authors whose scholarly work has enriched the intellectual foundation of this volume. Their rigorous research, interdisciplinary engagement, and commitment to advancing the fields of autonomous robotics, artificial intelligence, and healthcare innovation have been essential to the development of this book. We express our gratitude to the peer reviewers for their meticulous evaluations and constructive insights, which significantly enhanced the academic quality and coherence of the chapters. We also acknowledge the invaluable support provided by our respective institutions, whose academic environments and resources enabled us to undertake and complete this scholarly endeavor.

I extend my heartfelt gratitude to the Director of Vishwakarma Institute of Technology, Pune, for providing a supportive academic environment and for the continuous encouragement that made the development of this book, Revolutionizing Medicine with Autonomous Robotics, possible. I am equally thankful to the All Head of the Department and the All Dean for their invaluable guidance, motivation, and institutional support throughout this endeavour. Their commitment to academic excellence has greatly contributed to the successful completion of this work.

Our thanks are further extended to the editorial and production teams for their professionalism, editorial guidance, and consistent coordination throughout the publication process. Finally, we recognize the broader scientific and clinical communities whose pioneering work continues to inspire progress at the intersection of robotics, AI, and medicine. Their contributions form the foundation upon which *Revolutionizing Medicine with Autonomous Robotics* has been conceptualized and realized.

Chapter 1
Impact of NAMI Robots on Collision Detection, Avoidance, and Applications

Abhishek Kumar
https://orcid.org/0000-0003-3961-9970
Lovely Professional University, India

Harpreet Singh Bedi
https://orcid.org/0000-0003-1389-4333
Lovely Professional University, India

ABSTRACT

This chapter includes the implementation, applications, benefits, and potential of Navigational Autonomous Mapping Interface (NAMI) robots. NAMI robots, designed with advanced sensing, perception, and decision-making capabilities, utilize a combination of sensors, machine learning algorithms, and real-time data processing to improve their interaction with dynamic environments. It has a considerable impact on collision detection and collision avoidance into industrial application. The NAMI robot is a humanoid designed with multiple advances sensors and able to takes decision based on received sensor values to avoid collision. NAMI robots can explore unknown territories without causing damage to them. It proves to be a valuable tool for exploration and information support.

DOI: 10.4018/979-8-3373-0179-2.ch001

t © 2026, IGI Global Scientific Publishing. Copying or distributing in print or electronic forms without written permission of IGI Global Scientific Publishing is prohibited. Use of this chapter to
enerative artificial intelligence (AI) technologies is expressly prohibited. The publisher reserves all rights to license its use for generative AI training and machine learning model development.

1. INTRODUCTION

Humanoid robots like NAMI (Kitagawa et al. 2009) (Ogava N, 2020) are particularly remarkable among these advancements because they have the potential to provide engagement, rehabilitation, and ways that were previously only found in science fiction. Robots have gained significant importance in various industries and fields, including manufacturing, healthcare, agriculture, and logistics (Saadati 2023) (Cojocaru et al. 2022). One of the fundamental challenges in robots in the sports industry is enabling robots to navigate autonomously in complex and dynamic environments while avoiding obstacles. Obstacle avoidance is a critical aspect of autonomous robotics as it ensures the safety and efficiency of robot operations. An obstacle avoidance robot is a type of autonomous robot that can navigate through the environment with features of detection and avoidance of obstacles. To ensure smooth and secure mobility, these robots use a range of sensors, algorithms, and technologies that understand their environment and modify their path. Sports venues are often large, complex layout areas and unpredictable footfall. In these crowded areas, an autonomous obstacle-avoiding robot can recognize and maneuver around obstructions including people, furniture, sporting goods, and other environmental hazards.

The Navigational Autonomous Mapping Interface (N.A.M.I.) is an advancement in robot navigation that combines state-of-the-art technologies such as Simultaneous Localization and Mapping (SLAM), Lidar sensors, artificial intelligence (AI), and Robotic Operating System (ROS) to achieve previously levels of accuracy and efficiency. It assist robots, drones, or driverless cars in navigating a space by creating and employing precise maps. The system enables the device to make decisions in real time based on the map and environmental data, and these maps are generated automatically. The increasing desire for autonomous robots to function in dynamic and unexpected surroundings requires the development of advanced navigation systems that can adjust and respond in real time. N.A.M.I. is a cutting-edge robotic system designed for effective sports services facility management. N.A.M.I. improves the management of complicated sporting venues, such as stadiums and training facilities, by concurrently producing dynamic maps of its surroundings and pinpointing their exact location inside those maps. With its Lidar (Light Detection and Ranging) sensor, N.A.M.I. can detect and avoid obstacles by conducting 360-degree scans in real time. This ability is essential for guaranteeing seamless operations during events at busy sporting venues where prompt adjustments to shifting conditions are required. N.A.M.I. uses artificial intelligence (AI) tags as predefined destinations to increase navigation accuracy. By facilitating point-to-point movement, these tags allow the robot to guide spectators, help with maintenance duties, and deliver equipment efficiently. Tasks like organizing event areas, maintaining concession stand inventory, and performing regular facility equipment checks require this feature. NAMI enables the system to localize itself within the map while adjusting to dynamic changes in the surroundings by using advanced algorithms such as SLAM (Simultaneous Localization and Mapping). In order to ensure safe and effective navigation, it also integrates path planning and obstacle avoidance strategies, which makes it an essential technology in applications ranging from driverless cars to warehouse robots and agricultural equipment. The secret to NAMI's success in autonomous navigation is its capacity to combine sensor data and make decisions in real time using both static and dynamic information.

This chapter focuses on the development of an obstacle avoidance robot using Arduino, a versatile and widely accessible microcontroller platform (Pavitha et al., 2023) (Gomes et al, 2024) . The Robotic Operating System (ROS) serves as the foundation for the software framework that underpins N.A.M.I. and offers an adaptable platform for creating and incorporating complex robotic features. Based on Types of Navigation systems there are Behavior-based navigation systems and Model-based navigation systems (Tani 1996) (Na & Oh, 2023) (Yaonan et al 2011).

1.1. Behavior-Based Navigation System (Abascal et al., 2005)

A robotics approach presented in Figure 1 is a behavior-based navigation system that focuses on developing intelligent agents that can navigate diverse surroundings by applying easy-to-understand decentralized principles. Behavior-based navigation systems allow robots to react dynamically to their environment by imitating natural behaviors, in contrast to traditional navigation systems that rely on intricate algorithms or global maps (Antonelo, E. A., & Schrauwen, B. (2014). Behavior-based navigation systems operate under the premise that sensors and actuators are prone to noise and have limited information, leading them to avoid the creation of detailed geometric maps. The robot's behavior is governed by predefined rules. The robot's sensor architectures and the robotic control enable the robot to make decisions based on reactive behavior. Every behavior is a simple action or reaction to certain circumstances. For example, the robot may alter its speed or direction to avoid an obstruction if it detects one. The robot's control system uses real-time sensor inputs to decide which of these concurrent activities should be prioritized. As a result, these systems refrain from engaging in explicit reasoning about localization and position. Instead, they focus on crafting sets of behaviors that collaborate to accomplish the intended robot motion.

Figure 1. Behavior-based navigation system

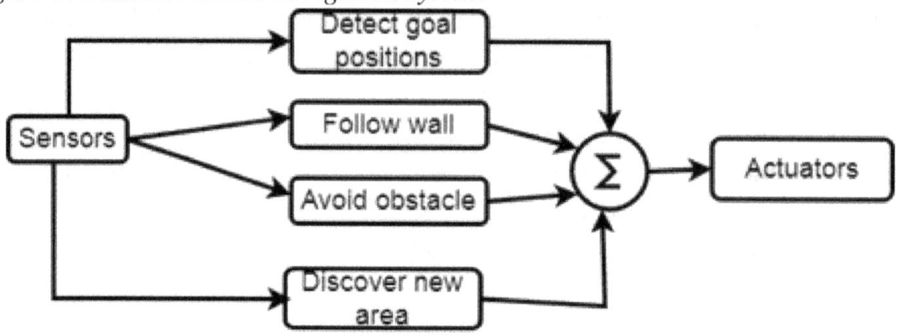

The following are the Key Features of the Behavior Navigation System (Fernandez-Leon et al, 2014)

1.1.1 Reactive Behavior

The focus of behavior-based navigation is on quick responses to outside cues. Instead of following pre-programmed routes, robots utilize sensors to sense their environment and react to impediments or changes in the ground (Bachelder, I. A., & Waxman, A. M. 1995). When a robot identifies a nearby object, it responds to local signals by slowing down, backing up, or turning away from obstacles. When the robot's sensors identify an obstruction, it may steer to the left or right. Unless a barrier is found, the robot may have a behavior that pushes it ahead toward a goal.

1.1.2 Modular Architecture

The system is organized in a modular way, allowing various behaviors (goal-seeking, obstacle avoidance, and exploration) to function both alone and together. This makes it possible to be adaptive and flexible in a variety of circumstances (Chiang, W., & Jin, Y. 2011).

1.1.3 Distributed Control

Behavior-based systems disperse decision-making over several behaviors as opposed to a central control unit. Because every activity has its own set of guidelines and priorities, the robot may navigate by taking a variety of aspects into account (Lau, H. Y., & Wong, V. W. 2007).

1.1.4 Learning and Adaptation

Some behavior-based systems have learning mechanisms built in, which allow robots to gradually get more effective at what they do by drawing on their past experiences and interactions with the environment (Sheridan, T. B. 2016).

1.1.5 Real-Time Decision

The robot makes judgments in real-time and on the fly with behavior-based systems; it eliminates the need for a complicated, predetermined plan. The robot can rapidly adjust to changes in its environment because of its dynamic decision-making mechanism.

1.1.6 Behavior Fusion and Priority

The robot may face multiple tasks, and some of the signals may take precedence over others. For example, if the robot notices an impending barrier in its path, it might prioritize obstacle avoidance over goal-seeking. Sometimes the robot can combine them in a way that produces coherent, effective action.

1.2. Model-Based Navigation System (Zhou & Wu, 2023)

An advanced kind of robotic navigation in Figure 2 is a model-based navigation system relying on an extensive internal representation, or model, of the surrounding environment. Model-based systems plan and carry out navigation tasks using structured information about their environment, in contrast to behavior-based systems, which concentrate on reactive responses. A model-based navigation system is a kind of robotic navigation that plans and regulates movement using internal models of the robot's surroundings. In contrast to behavior-based systems, which focus on real-time responses to sensor data, a model-based system plans and predicts the best routes before the robot moves, frequently using complex algorithms and computational methods to navigate and avoid obstacles. It allows robots to function well in intricate situations by allowing them to make judgments based on prior knowledge as well as current sensory information. Model-based navigation systems explicitly employ the concept of position. No matter how complicated an environment is, they can adapt to it as long as they have accurate maps of the relevant environments (Joo, S. H et al. 2020).

Figure 2. Model-based navigation system

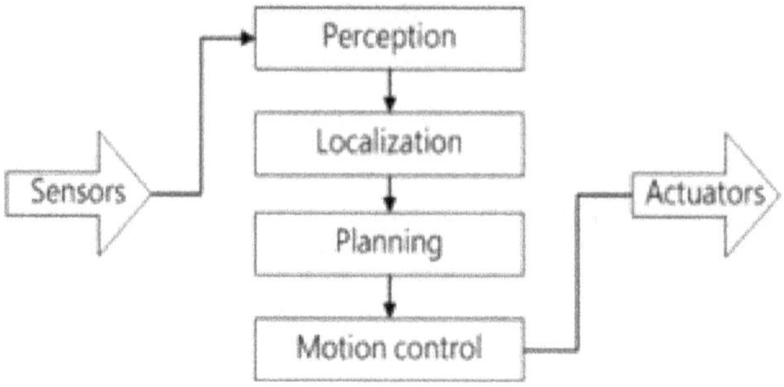

The following are the Key Features of a Model-based Navigation System (Raikwar, S., Fehrmann, J., & Herlitzius, T. 2022)

1.2.1 Environmental Modeling

With the use of geometric, topological, and semantic data, these systems generate detailed maps or models of the surroundings. Robots can navigate and understand spatial relationships. The map is either pre-loaded or built dynamically as the robot explores, using sensors like LIDAR, cameras, and ultrasonic sensors to gather data and update the model in real-time.

1.2.2 Path Planning

Robots can choose the best way from a starting point to a destination by using algorithms for path planning, which are frequently used in model-based navigation, might involve using Dijkstra's, A, or Rapidly Exploring Random Trees (RRT) algorithms. An ideal path from the robot's current location to its goal while avoiding known obstacles is determined using global path planning algorithms (A* or Dijkstra's algorithm). These algorithms determine the optimal route by taking into account several variables, including barriers, distance, and energy efficiency.

1.2.3 Position Estimation

The robot needs to be able to estimate its position correctly relative to the map. This is accomplished by localization in which the robot maps its environment and records its location on that map. As it moves, the robot can update its position. The robot must simultaneously modify its trajectory locally in response to real-time sensor inputs. For example, if an obstacle suddenly appears, the robot may temporarily modify its path to avoid the obstacle but will return to its global path once the obstacle is passed (Vatavu, A. et al, 2020)

1.2.4 Integration of Sensor Input

To update their internal models and increase navigation accuracy, model-based systems combine input from a variety of sensors (LIDAR, cameras, and IMUs) (Yang, M. et al, 2022). The robot uses sensor feedback to identify any unexpected obstructions as it travels along the predetermined route. The robot can (a) Recalculate a new path that avoids the obstacle based on the environment model (b) change its speed and (c) direction until the barrier is away from its path.

Figure 3. Developing process of mobile robot global/reactive path planning

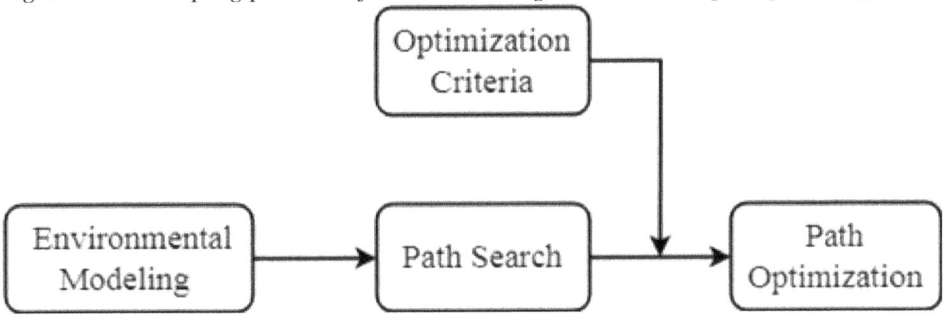

Mobile robot path planning is a crucial aspect of robotic navigation, allowing robots to move efficiently and safely through their environments. The development of global and reactive path planning involves a structured process that integrates various algorithms, sensor data, and environmental models. The block diagram in Figure 3 includes algorithm selection, real-time changes, and environmental modeling are involved in the development of mobile robot global and reactive path planning. An extensive environment map is made utilizing different methods like geometric maps or grid mapping, including sensor integration for data collecting in real-time. Reactive paths use feedback loops from sensors to identify changing obstacles and modify the robot's direction accordingly. By using methods such as behavior-based control or potential fields, the robot may react instantly to changes in its environment. By utilizing a hybrid strategy that integrates the benefits of global and reactive planning, the robot can effectively negotiate intricate settings. Lastly, performance evaluation and optimization are carried out. Metrics like success rate, path length, and reaction time are evaluated to improve the navigation system's resilience and dependability for practical uses.

2. IMPLEMENTATION OF NAMI ROBOT

The NAMI robot was developed with navigation features (Polydoros, A. S., & Nalpantidis, L. 2017). Incorporating Autonomous Mobile Robots into sports services is a step toward more effective facility management. This deliberate action responds to the increasing demand for improved reactivity and streamlined operations in contemporary sporting venues, such as training centers and stadiums. Mobile Robots are made to function independently, doing duties that normally call for human assistance. Advanced sensors, powerful data processing power, and navigation systems enable this independence (He, D. Q., Wang, H. B., & Li, P. F. 2018). Robots can gather and examine enormous volumes of environmental data by using technologies such as Lidar, cameras, and Inertial Measurement Units (IMUs), which enables them to navigate intricate layouts, comprehend their environment, and avoid obstacles in real time. Mobile robots can optimize a variety of logistical responsibilities in sports facility administration. They are capable of managing concession stand inventory, moving equipment between locations, and helping with venue maintenance, for instance. Their capacity to function effectively in hectic settings ensures that events run without any problems, enhancing the experience for athletes and spectators.

The NAMI robot's obstacle-detecting characteristics and left and right-moving skills are very helpful on industrial application. The robot helps industrial person evasive maneuvers and decision-making, by replicating unpredictable circumstances. Humance being can improve their reaction speeds and make faster decisions in real-world scenarios by utilizing this interaction (Miao, Z., & Ge, G. 2023). Furthermore, by modifying its speed and complexity according to the athlete's performance, the robot may offer customized training that fosters the development of specific skills. By refining their techniques in a controlled environment, athletes can train with the NAMI robot and lower their chance of injury from erroneous motions. Moreover, coaches can evaluate athletes' interactions and give tailored feedback using the data gathered by the robot's sensors, improving training results. Overall the NAMI robot is a useful tool for enhancing athletic performance, boosting self-esteem, and educating athletes about the dynamics of competition (Robot, M. 2024) (Baur, K et al, 2018) (Evripidou, S at al, 2020).

Figure 4. Block diagram of interfaced mobile diagram

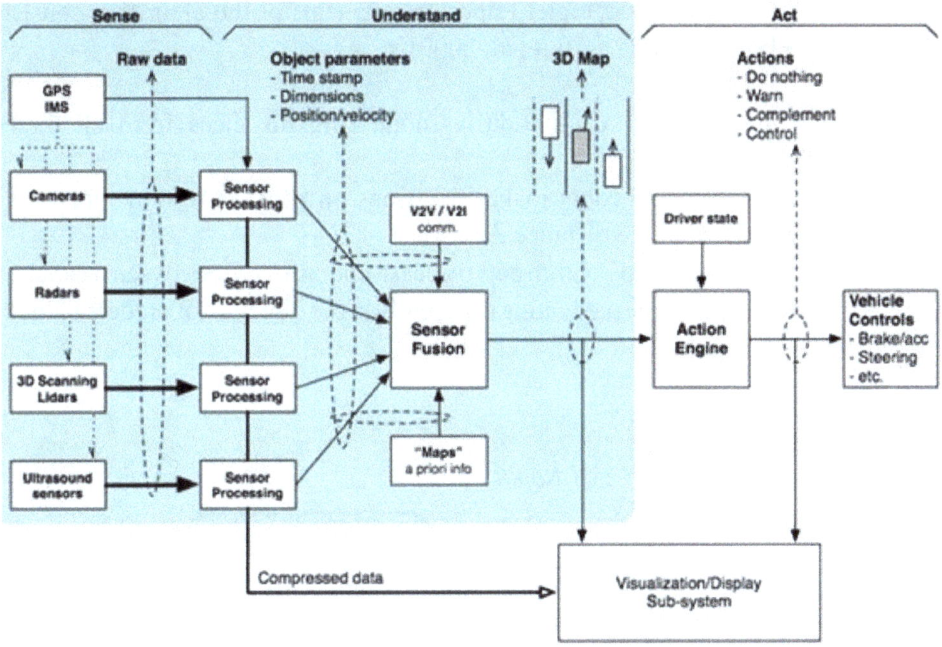

Figure 4 presents the block diagram of the interfaced NAMI mobile robot. NAMI utilizes three ultrasonic distance sensors to detect obstacles by measuring the distances to surrounding objects. By combining three ultrasonic distance sensors, the NAMI robot project seeks to improve obstacle recognition and navigational skills. The robot was originally just intended to have one sensor, but the inclusion of two more greatly enhances its capacity to recognize impediments in its surroundings, which in turn improves its autonomous navigational abilities. The robot is programmed using Arduino software and runs on an Arduino Microcontroller platform. The idea may be replicated and modified thanks to the user-friendly approach made possible by the selection of hardware and software. The three ultrasonic distance sensors must work together to provide complete coverage and remove blind areas that have historically led to navigational collisions. The robot's left, right, and front are all covered by the three ultrasonic sensors that are placed carefully. Because of its arrangement, the robot has fewer blind spots and can detect impediments in all directions. By sending out ultrasonic waves and timing the return of the echoes, each sensor determines how far away from adjacent objects it is. The robot can make navigation decisions in real-time by processing this data to estimate the closeness of obstacles. The navigation algorithm has been developed to ensure movement without collisions while keeping the journey distance to a minimum. A flowchart in Figure 5 that shows how the robot interprets sensor data and reacts to barriers it detects visually represents the logic. Important elements of the algorithm consist of (Mateus et al, 2024) (Bideau, B.,et al, 2009)

A) *Obstacle Identification:* Continuously monitoring distances from all three sensors.
B) *Making Decisions:* The robot makes decisions on whether to move forward, turn, or halt based on the distance data.
C) *Path Optimization*: The algorithm puts the least amount of time between obstacles and the destination while navigating efficiently in the direction of predetermined milestones.

Figure 5. Flowchart of the NAMI Robot

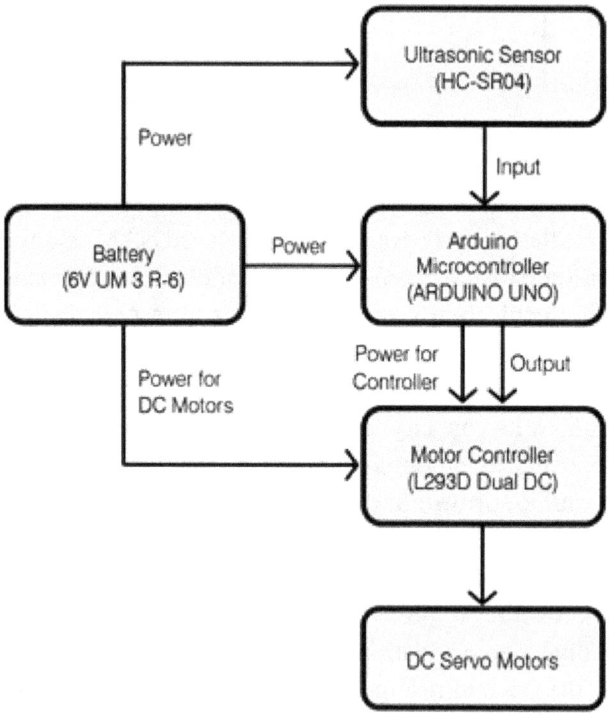

The robot's primary objective is to identify any object within a predetermined threshold distance (Sezer, V., & Gokasan, M. 2012) (Kumar, A. 2024). When an object is detected within this range, it is classified as an obstacle, prompting the robot to change its course away from it. The robot features three ultrasonic sensors positioned at the front section—right, middle, and left, presented in Figure 6. These sensors emit ultrasonic pulses every 300 milliseconds and these pulses bounce off nearby objects. Using the time difference between sending the pulse and receiving the echo, Arduino calculates the distance to the obstacle based on the constant speed of sound at 340 m/s. If one of the sensors detects an obstacle within the threshold distance, the robot alters its direction accordingly. In addition to these fundamental movements, the robot is designed to address more intricate scenarios where all three sensors detect obstacles within the specified range. In such instances, the robot briefly moves backward for 10 milliseconds and then re-evaluates the distances to objects using the right and left sensors. Subsequently, the robot compares these two distances and moves in the direction where the distance is greater.

Figure 6. Obstacle Avoiding Algorithm for Robot

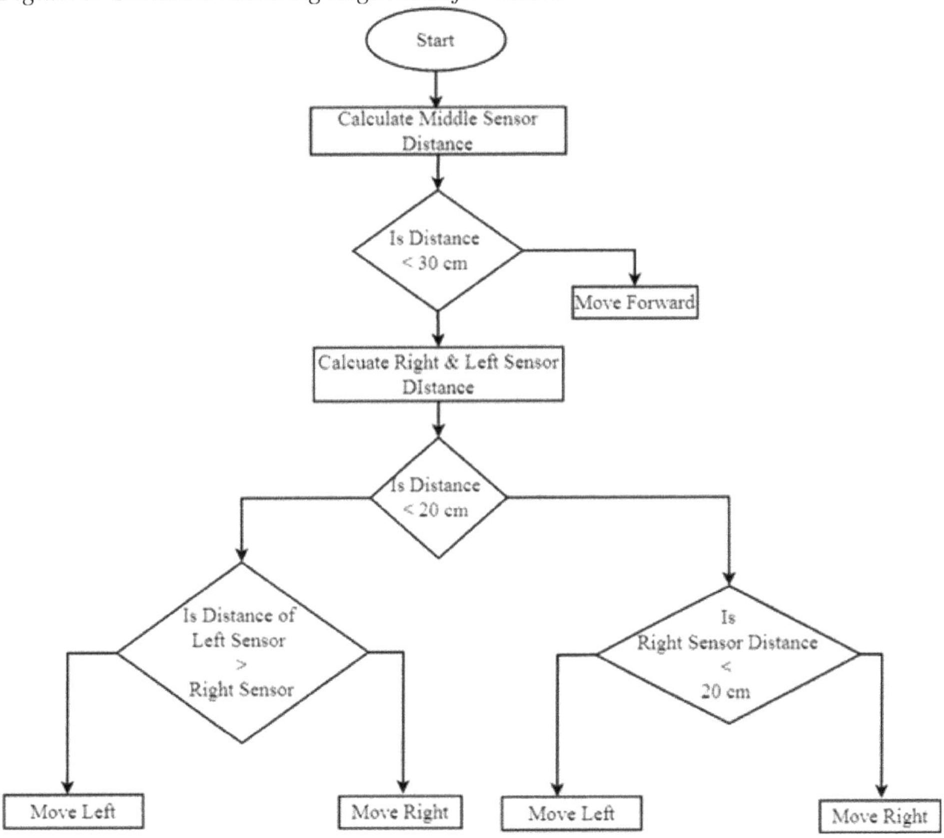

2.1 Hardware Components of NAMI Robot

The NAMI robot is constructed using a combination of essential hardware components that work together to facilitate its autonomous navigation and obstacle-detection capabilities. These hardware elements, which include an Arduino Uno, motor drivers, ultrasonic sensors, a motorized chassis, and a rechargeable battery, provide a strong basis for the NAMI robot. When combined, they allow the robot to explore its surroundings on its own and recognize and avoid obstacles with efficiency. This construction not only shows how well robotics design concepts work but also emphasizes how easily accessible the parts are for learning and growth.

2.1.1 The Uno Arduino

The NAMI robot's central control unit is the Arduino Uno. It performs the control algorithms that specify how the robot moves by processing data from the ultrasonic sensors. The Uno is a great option for robotics projects because of its adaptability and simplicity of programming.

2.1.2 Sound Absorption Sensors

The HC-SR04 ultrasonic sensors that are installed on the robot are essential for determining distances and identifying obstructions. Robotic systems that must work in tight places depend on these sensors' capability to measure distances, which is especially helpful in close-range. The HC-SR04 measures the time it takes for ultrasonic waves to return after striking an object after they have been emitted. The system can then detect objects and modify its trajectory by converting this time into a distance measurement. The integration of these sensors into the NAMI framework enhances the system's capability to detect obstacles and make precise adjustments in real-time, ensuring smoother navigation and preventing collisions in dynamic or cluttered environments.

2.1.3 DC Motor and Motor Drivers

DC is used for the locomotion of the AMR. Each motor typically drives one wheel, allowing for basic movements such as forward, backward, and turning. The robot's wheels are driven by two DC motors that are controlled by L298N motor drivers. Based on the control signals received from the Arduino, the motor drivers regulate the motors' speed and direction. This part is essential to the robot's ability to move about its surroundings.

2.1.4 Wheels and Chassis

The basic chassis of the NAMI robot holds the components and offers structural support. For stability, there are two driven wheels in addition to a roller wheel. During navigation, this posture enables balance and fluid movement.

2.1.5 RPLIDAR

RoboPeak developed RPLIDAR, a flexible, reasonably priced 360-degree laser scanner that is utilized in applications requiring accurate mapping, obstacle identification, and distance measuring. This scanner uses revolving laser beams to quickly and accurately collect data from its surroundings, creating intricate 2D point cloud maps of the surroundings. RPLIDAR estimates distances to different barriers or objects by using a laser source, range finder, and a rotating motor. By measuring the time it takes for a laser beam to reach an object and return, it works on the Time-of-Flight (TOF) principle, enabling precise distance measurements over a range of distances. RPLIDAR is capable of gathering thousands of data points at a scanning frequency of up to 8000 times per second, with a rotational speed of about 4000 revolutions per minute (RPM) and a scanning range of up to 8 meters (Raj, T et al 2020). The scanner can be easily integrated with a wide range of platforms and devices, including robots, drones, and autonomous cars, thanks to its many connection options, which include USB, UART, and I2C. Its lightweight and small form makes it simple to install and use in a variety of applications. RPLIDAR has multiple scanning modes, such as targeted scanning for faster data collection in particular regions of interest and full 360-degree scanning for thorough environmental mapping. Additionally, it has sophisticated features including multi-scanning mode, which enables simultaneous scanning with multiple RPLIDAR units for improved range and density, and adaptive scanning, which modifies the scanning frequency based on object distance. RPLIDAR also includes a software development kit (SDK) that offers developers a comprehensive collection of tools and APIs to incorporate the scanner into their apps. It is very compatible and accessible to a broad spectrum of developers and consumers because it supports well-known software platforms including ROS, Arduino, and Raspberry Pi. Because of its adaptability, RPLIDAR is a crucial instrument for robotics, mapping, and environmental sensing applications. In Figure 7 sensor has a laser beam that is turned on and off according to a predetermined frequency or pattern is called a modulated laser pulse. The sensor can coordinate the timing of the emitted pulse with the anticipated return time of reflected pulses because the RPLIDAR emits these modulated pulses in quick succession. This synchronization reduces interference from outside light sources and improves measurement accuracy. The emitted pulse returns to the sensor as a reflected pulse when it comes into contact with a boundary, like a surface or object. Accurately determining the distance to the border depends on the time of this return pulse, which also helps with mapping and obstacle identification in the surrounding area.

Figure 7. Working module of RPLIDAR sensor

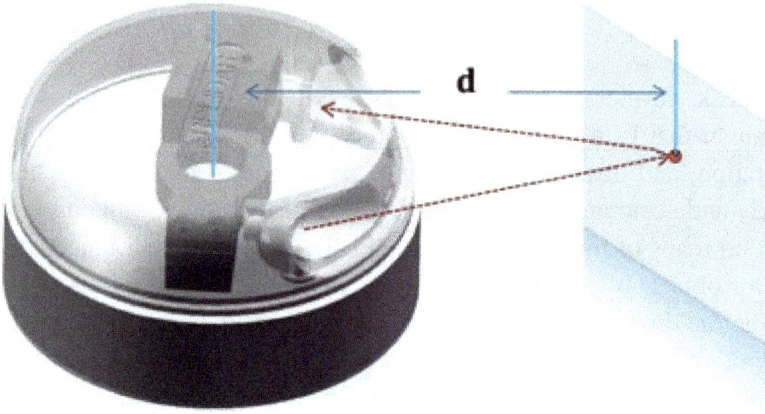

Sourc: Pereira Mendes and Lim (2024)

2.16. Power Source

Rechargeable Li-ion batteries provide a portable and effective energy source for the robot. This battery is suitable since it can run for longer periods and is simple to replenish.

2.2 Software Components of the NAMI Robot

The NAMI robot's software architecture is designed to enable effective programming, navigation, and control of the robot's movements. The software components of the NAMI robot, including the Arduino IDE, C/C++ programming, a custom obstacle avoidance algorithm, and PID control, collectively enable effective autonomous navigation and obstacle detection.

2.2.1 The Arduino IDE

The primary device for programming the Arduino Uno microcontroller is the Arduino Integrated Development Environment (IDE). The IDE makes it easy to write, compile, and upload code to the Arduino board, allowing for simple software testing and development for the robot.

2.2.2 Programming in C/C++

C/C++ code is utilized to control the robot's actions. With the performance and control required for hardware interfaces, this programming language is ideal for embedded systems. The robot's autonomous functions are made possible by the efficient processing of sensor data and the execution of complicated algorithms made possible by the usage of C/C++.

2.2.3 Obstacle Avoidance Algorithm

An obstacle avoidance algorithm is implemented to process the data received from the ultrasonic sensors. This algorithm continuously analyzes distance measurements to detect obstacles and make real-time navigation decisions.

A) Identifying obstacles based on sensor readings.
B) Determining appropriate maneuvers (stopping, turning) to avoid collisions.
C) Ensuring smooth navigation while maintaining a minimum distance from obstacles.

The obstacle avoidance algorithm follows.

A) *Sensor Data Acquisition:* Ultrasonic sensors continuously measure the distances to obstacles in front of the robot.
B) *Data Processing:* The collected distance data are processed to determine the presence and proximity of obstacles.
C) *Decision Making:* Based on the sensor data, the robot decides whether to move forward, turn left, turn right, or stop.
D) *Motor Control: The* motor drivers are used to control the speed and direction of the robot's wheels to execute the chosen action. Hardware Components and Assembly hardware used to build the robot and explain the relationship (input and output) among them.
E) *PID Control:* To accomplish accurate and steady motions, the robot utilizes a Proportional-Integral-Derivative (PID) control mechanism. The robot can respond to different inputs more precisely, which enables it to dynamically change its direction and speed. During navigation, the PID controller aids in preserving stability, especially while making turns or reacting to abrupt environmental changes.

The use of software enables adaptable behavior, ensuring the robot's ability to function effectively in constantly shifting circumstances without running into obstacles. These characteristics serve as a basis for future improvements and alterations in addition to demonstrating the NAMI robot's capabilities.

4. RESULT AND DISCUSSION

The Robotic Operating System (ROS) and Gazebo were used to mimic an environment in which the NAMI robot was subjected to intensive testing. These techniques reduced development risks and expenses by enabling the construction of a controlled, virtual environment where the robot could be put through rigorous testing without the need for actual trials. Because the simulation environment mimicked real-world conditions, it was possible to test navigation techniques, obstacle identification, and reaction to environmental changes. Assessing the NAMI system's ability to recognize and steer clear of obstacles using its sensors and algorithms in a range of situations was the primary objective. The simulation's results and conclusions are presented in this section, with an emphasis on obstacle identification and navigational practices. To replicate real-world settings for the NAMI robot, an online environment was built for the ROS Gazebo simulation environment and Unity simulation environment shown in Figure 8. In this setting, two robots equipped with laser sensors capable of detecting obstacles and navigating around them. The NAMI interface was used to train these robots, which used a combination of path-planning algorithms, sensor fusion, and laser-based SLAM to explore the area on their own. Particularly important to obstacle recognition were the laser sensors, which enabled the robot to gauge the separation between objects in its path and modify its trajectory to prevent collisions.

Figure 8. (A) Gazebo training environment (B) Gazebo testing environment (C) Unity training environment (D) Unity testing environment (E) Raw camera image (F) Statically labeled image (G) Object of interest

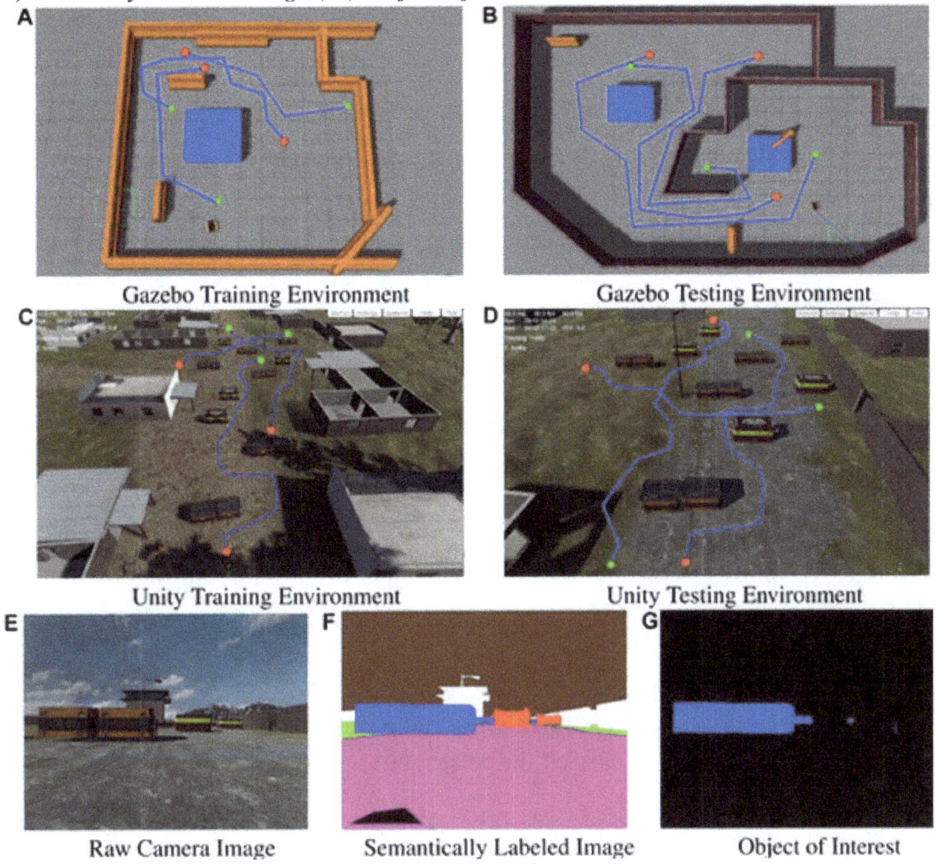

The configuration enables a controlled setting and dynamic testing of the robot's navigation algorithms. Based on data obtained from the laser grid, the robots are designed to react when they identify an obstacle:

4.1. Laser Beam Detection

Every robot has a laser sensor installed that forms a grid to measure distances. The leftmost and rightmost areas of the divided grid are critical for navigational decisions.

4.2 Turning Behaviour

The robot is designed to turn right if it detects an obstruction in the leftmost grid. In contrast, the robot will turn left if it detects an obstruction in the rightmost grid.

4.3 Odd Number of Grids

To make navigation logic simpler, the decision-making procedure employs an odd number of grids. The robot will pivot to the side with less damaged grids when it detects an impediment in the middle of its body, improving its response to obstacles.

4.4 Straight-Line Following

The robots are made to stay on a straight path when there are no obstructions in their way, which makes for effective environmental navigation.

4.5 Display of Information

The ROS command console provides pertinent information during the simulation. This result consists of:

- Obstacle detection state.
- The trajectory and current position of the robot.
- Instructions are being carried out in response to sensor data.

This feedback is essential for monitoring the robot's behavior and troubleshooting any issues that arise during simulation. The ability to visualize this process in a simulated world not only validates the robot's design but also serves as a valuable tool for future development and optimization.

Figure 9. Movement of Robot moving forward.

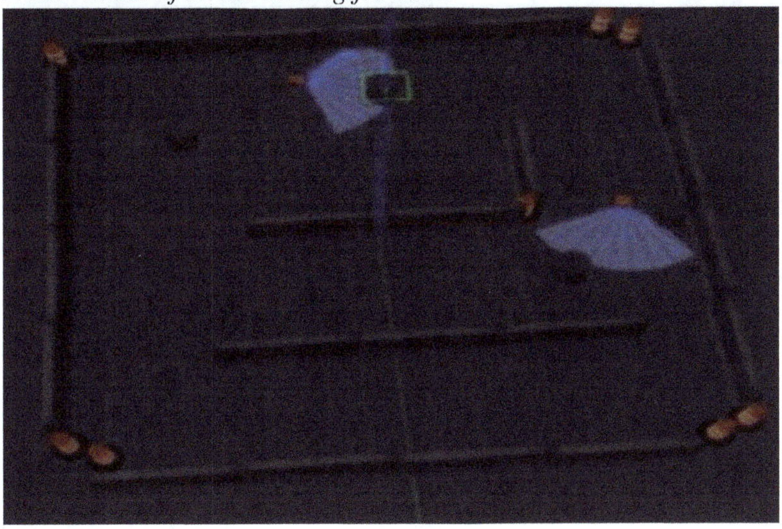

Figure 9 presents the robot moving forward, the laser grid detecting walls so the robot will turn opposite the direction until grids become light blue, then the robot will move forward. The grid turns from light blue to a more vivid color (signaling a possible collision) when the robot senses an obstruction. Once the impediment has been successfully avoided, the robot automatically spins in the opposite direction until the laser grid lightens to a bright blue color once more. Clear space is indicated by the grid's bright blue hue, which permits the robot to continue moving forward. Effective obstacle avoidance is ensured by this feedback loop, in which the robot continuously adapts in response to color changes in the grid. presents both robots moving forward they are detecting no obstacle because both laser grids are light blue. The laser grids of both robots show light blue in this situation, suggesting that the way forward is unobstructed. The robots are able to travel steadily and continuously since there are no barriers in their way. The simulation's a position of two robots provides light on how the system manages several agents moving through the same area where robots must communicate with one another while avoiding obstacles.

Figure 10. Movement of Robot detecting no obstacle

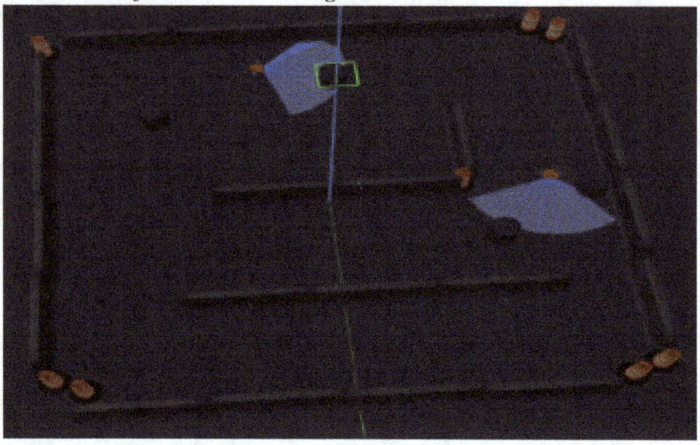

Figure 11. Detection of obstacle Detecting the obstacle close enough and less grid line is dark.

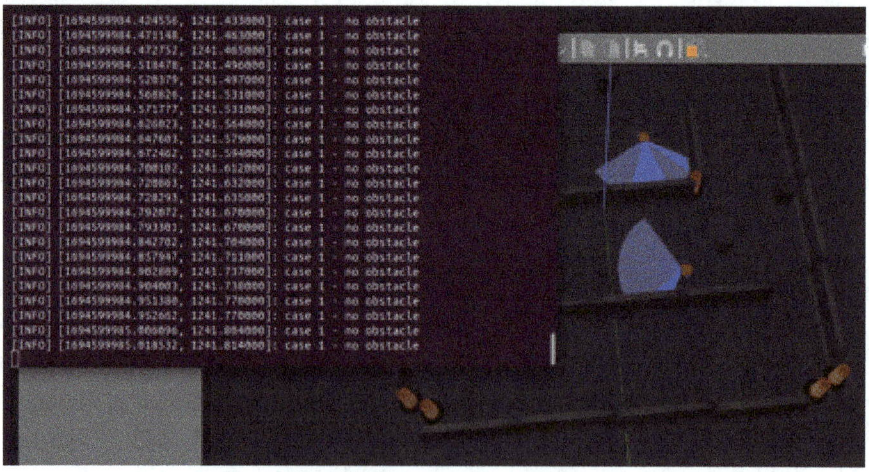

Figure 12. Detection of obstacle at front and wall at the left.

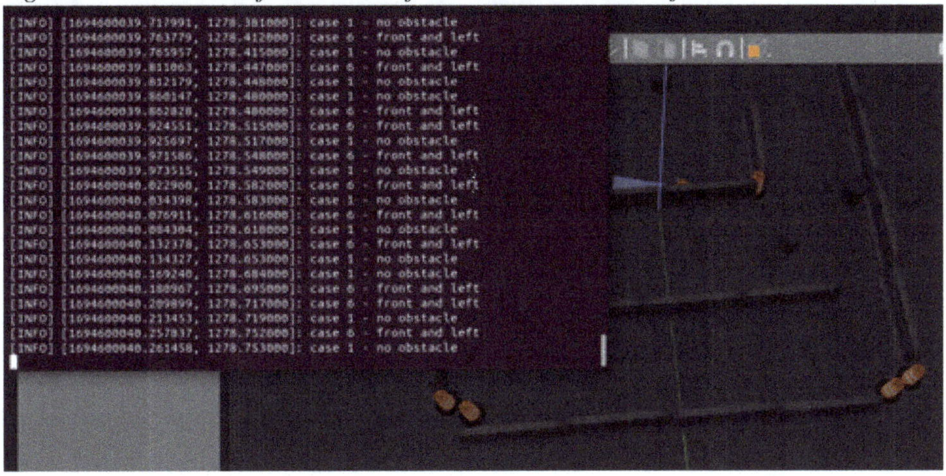

The command console gives an accurate representation of the robot's performance and obstacle detection while providing real-time feedback about its surroundings and condition. Engineers and developers can track how the robot reacts to different stimuli, such obstacles and environmental changes, by examining the feedback from the command interface. This is essential for optimizing the robot's navigation algorithms. shows the command terminal showing no obstacle because both robots not detecting the obstacle close enough and fewer grid lines are dark. The command console indicates that neither robot has spotted any nearby obstacles when both robots are proceeding without running into any. On the robots' interfaces, the laser grids show up as light blue, signifying that the way ahead is clear. The fewer dark grid lines—which are usually used to indicate detected obstacles—reflect this trend. Light blue indicates that there are no obstacles in the way, so the robots can continue on their path undisturbed. In the command terminal, this status might be displayed with a message like:

> "**Robot 1:** No obstacles detected. Path clear."
> "**Robot 2:** No obstacles detected. Path clear."

Both robots can proceed forward without needing to change their course because the terminal displays few dark grid lines, indicating that the laser system hasn't detected any nearby obstacles. This is perfect for uninterrupted, effective navigation, which is crucial in settings where quick mobility is necessary, like obstacle courses. When the environment is clear, the robots can move freely and make quick decisions because they can only detect obstacles when they are close enough. The command terminal displays a more complex interaction when one robot recognizes an obstacle while the other does not. Robot 1's laser grid stays light blue in this situation, signifying that there are no obstructions in its way. Robot 2, on the other hand, detects an impediment ahead when its grid turns dark red or another color. As the technology detects the obstacle's closeness, the grid lines in this area get darker. The command terminal in shows one robot detecting no obstacle and another one detecting obstacle at the front and wall at the left.

The terminal display the following message

"**Robot 1:** No obstacles detected. Path clear."
"**Robot 2:** Obstacle detected at front. Wall detected on the left."

Feedback shows that Robot 2 has come across a scenario in which a wall on the left side and an impediment in front of it are both present, causing the system to act. Robot 2 will probably change its trajectory in response to the laser grid readings, either veering to the right to avoid the wall on the left or turning away from the barrier in front. A clear visual depiction of Robot 2's decision-making process is provided by the increasing quantity of dark grid lines on the interface, which show how the system detects nearby obstacles. The command terminal's response is essential for understanding how the robot adjusts to obstacles. When the terminal detects that Robot 2 is approaching an obstruction, it starts to modify its motion and speed accordingly, based on the obstacles' proximity, to prevent collisions.

3. ADVANTAGE AND LIMITATION

3.1 The NAMI Robot Offers the Following Advantages

1. The NAMI robot can be used in fields such as urban planning, disaster response, and robotics training.
2. The robot's real-time feedback capabilities are invaluable for educational, professional, or personal development goals.
3. The NAMI robot's ability to recognize obstacles can be used in settings like building sites, industrial sites, or even risky rescue operations where people's safety is a top priority.
4. Because the robot can mimic real-world interactions, it can be used in situations when quick decisions are needed, such emergency response, military training, or even healthcare simulation.
5. Robots' captivating and interactive technology can boost motivation.

3.2 The NAMI Robot Has Many Advantages for Sports Training, But It Has Limitations

1. Although they can carry out some activities or simulate situations, robots frequently find it difficult to capture the dynamic and unpredictable nature of real-world settings.
2. It can be costly to build and maintain high-quality robots with sophisticated features.
3. The design and technology of robots frequently limit their range of motion.
4. The development of important human abilities like problem-solving, critical thinking, and fast decision-making may be hampered by the ongoing usage of robots in operational or training environments.
5. All machines, including robots, eventually wear out. Their frequent maintenance requirements and possible malfunctions may cause disruptions to everyday operations, job procedures, or training plans.
6. Robots can be trained to recognize barriers and follow predetermined routes, but they may find it difficult to adjust to more complex or uncertain circumstances.

4. CONCLUSION

The use of robotics in sports training has advanced significantly with the introduction of the NAMI robot. Athletes have access to a distinct platform for improved practice and skill development because of its left and right movement capabilities and advanced obstacle identification. The robot helps athletes refine their reaction speeds, polish their techniques, and gain confidence in navigating unpredictable surroundings by imitating real-world events. Its effectiveness is further enhanced by the capacity to personalize training programs according to each individual's performance, enabling a customized approach to skill improvement. In addition, the information gathered from the robot's interactions provides trainers with insightful information that helps with focused criticism and ongoing development. Overall the NAMI robot is a useful and innovative tool that not only improves athletic performance but also encourages safety and injury prevention, making it a crucial component of contemporary sports training.

Acknowledgments

The authors would like to acknowledge the Robotics Lab or providing the facility to conduct the simulation work.

Conflicts of Interest: The authors declare no conflict of interest.

REFERENCES

Abascal, J., Lazkano, E., & Sierra, B. (2005). Behavior-based indoor navigation. Ambient Intelligence for Scientific Discovery: Foundations, Theories, and Systems, 263-285.

Antonelo, E. A., & Schrauwen, B. (2014). On learning navigation behaviors for small mobile robots with reservoir computing architectures. *IEEE Transactions on Neural Networks and Learning Systems*, *26*(4), 763–780. PMID: 25794381

Bachelder, I. A., & Waxman, A. M. (1995). A view-based neurocomputational system for relational map-making and navigation in visual environments. *Robotics and Autonomous Systems*, *16*(2-4), 267–289.

Baur, K., Schättin, A., de Bruin, E. D., Riener, R., Duarte, J. E., & Wolf, P. (2018). Trends in robot-assisted and virtual reality-assisted neuromuscular therapy: A systematic review of health-related multiplayer games. *Journal of Neuroengineering and Rehabilitation*, *15*, 1–19. PMID: 30454009

Bideau, B., Kulpa, R., Vignais, N., Brault, S., Multon, F., & Craig, C. (2009). Using virtual reality to analyze sports performance. *IEEE Computer Graphics and Applications*, *30*(2), 14–21. PMID: 20650707

Chiang, W., & Jin, Y. (2011, January). Toward a meta-model of behavioral interaction for designing complex adaptive systems. In *International Design Engineering Technical Conferences and Computers and Information in Engineering Conference* (Vol. 54792, pp. 1077-1088).

Cojocaru, A. M., Bucea-Manea- oni , R., Jianu, A., Dumangiu, M. A., Alexandrescu, L. U., & Cojocaru, M. (2022). The role of physical education and sports in modern society supported by IoT—A student perspective. *Sustainability*, *14*(9), 5624.

Evripidou, S., Georgiou, K., Doitsidis, L., Amanatiadis, A. A., Zinonos, Z., & Chatzichristofis, S. A. (2020). Educational robotics: Platforms, competitions and expected learning outcomes. *IEEE Access : Practical Innovations, Open Solutions*, *8*, 219534–219562.

Fernandez-Leon, J. A., Acosta, G. G., & Rozenfeld, A. (2014). How simple autonomous decisions evolve into robust behaviours?: A review from neurorobotics, cognitive, self-organized and artificial immune systems fields. *Bio Systems*, *124*, 7–20. PMID: 25149273

Gomes, R., Carmo, T., Braga, K., Santos, A., Andrade, C., & Andrade, E. (2024). Arduino programming of an educational robotic platform applied in radiological accident simulation. *Brazilian Journal of Radiation Sciences*, *12*(1), e2395–e2395.

He, D. Q., Wang, H. B., & Li, P. F. (2018, May). Robot path planning using improved rapidly-exploring random tree algorithm. In 2018 IEEE Industrial Cyber-Physical Systems (ICPS) (pp. 181-186). IEEE.

Joo, S. H., Manzoor, S., Rocha, Y. G., Bae, S. H., Lee, K. H., Kuc, T. Y., & Kim, M. (2020). Autonomous navigation framework for intelligent robots based on a semantic environment modeling. *Applied Sciences (Basel, Switzerland)*, *10*(9), 3219.

Kitagawa, Y., Ishikura, T., Song, W., Mae, Y., Minami, M., & Tanaka, K. (2009, August). Human-like patient robot with chaotic emotion for injection training. In 2009 ICCAS-SICE (pp. 4635-4640). IEEE.

Kumar, A. (2024). IoT-Enhanced Spy Robotics Bridging Security Gaps. In Shaping the Future of Automation With Cloud-Enhanced Robotics (pp. 343-358). IGI Global.

Lau, H. Y., & Wong, V. W. (2007). An immunity approach to strategic behavioral control. *Engineering Applications of Artificial Intelligence*, *20*(3), 289–306.

Mateus, N., Abade, E., Coutinho, D., Gómez, M. Á., Peñas, C. L., & Sampaio, J. (2024). Empowering the Sports Scientist with Artificial Intelligence in Training, Performance, and Health Management. *Sensors (Basel)*, *25*(1), 139. PMID: 39796930

Miao, Z., & Ge, G. (2023). Research on the Development of Sports in the Age of Artificial Intelligence. power, 5(7), 6-11.

Na, Y. K., & Oh, S. Y. (2003). Hybrid control for autonomous mobile robot navigation using neural network based behavior modules and environment classification. *Autonomous Robots*, *15*, 193–206.

Pavitha, N., Dardige, R., Patil, V., Pawar, A., & Shah, B. (2023, December). Obstacle Detection Using Arduino Board and Bluetooth Control. In International Conference on Information and Communication Technology for Competitive Strategies (pp. 297-307). Singapore: Springer Nature Singapore.

Pereira Mendes, C., & Lim, N. T. L. (2024). EcoLiDAR: An economical LiDAR scanner for ecological research. *PLoS One*, *19*(6), e0298712. PMID: 38917132

Polydoros, A. S., & Nalpantidis, L. (2017). Survey of model-based reinforcement learning: Applications on robotics. *Journal of Intelligent & Robotic Systems*, *86*(2), 153–173.

Raikwar, S., Fehrmann, J., & Herlitzius, T. (2022). Navigation and control development for a four-wheel-steered mobile orchard robot using model-based design. *Computers and Electronics in Agriculture*, *202*, 107410.

Raj, T., Hanim Hashim, F., Baseri Huddin, A., Ibrahim, M. F., & Hussain, A. (2020). A survey on LiDAR scanning mechanisms. *Electronics (Basel)*, *9*(5), 741.

Robot, M. (2024). Discourse analysis and communication strategy of sport learning: a systematic review assisted with VOSviewer. Retos: nuevas tendencias en educación física, deporte y recreación, (61), 430-439.

Saadati, S. A. (2023). Recent innovations in sports physiology: Shaping the future of athletic performance. *Health Nexus*, *1*(2), 15–27.

Sezer, V., & Gokasan, M. (2012). A novel obstacle avoidance algorithm:"Follow the Gap Method". *Robotics and Autonomous Systems*, *60*(9), 1123–1134.

Sheridan, T. B. (2016). Human–robot interaction: Status and challenges. *Human Factors*, *58*(4), 525–532. PMID: 27098262

Tani, J. (1996). Model-based learning for mobile robot navigation from the dynamical systems perspective. *IEEE Transactions on Systems, Man, and Cybernetics. Part B, Cybernetics*, *26*(3), 421–436. PMID: 18263044

Vatavu, A., Rahm, M., Govindachar, S., Krehl, G., Mantha, A., Bhavsar, S. R., & Maile, M. (2020). From particles to self-localizing tracklets: A multilayer particle filter-based estimation for dynamic grid maps. *IEEE Intelligent Transportation Systems Magazine*, *12*(4), 149–168.

Yang, M., Sun, X., Jia, F., Rushworth, A., Dong, X., Zhang, S., & Liu, B. (2022). Sensors and sensor fusion methodologies for indoor odometry: A review. *Polymers*, *14*(10), 2019. PMID: 35631899

Yaonan, W., Yimin, Y., Xiaofang, Y., Yi, Z., Yuanli, Z., Feng, Y., & Lei, T. (2011). Autonomous mobile robot navigation system designed in dynamic environment based on transferable belief model. *Measurement*, *44*(8), 1389–1405.

Zhou, R., & Wu, F. (2023). Inheritance and Innovation Development of Sports based on Deep Learning and Artificial Intelligence. *IEEE Access : Practical Innovations, Open Solutions*, *11*, 116511–116523.

Chapter 2
AI in Patient Monitoring

Yameen Liyakat Hakim
https://orcid.org/0000-0002-3187-1787
RIMT University, Punjab, India

Sushil Bhardwaj
https://orcid.org/0000-0001-5184-3866
RIMT University, Punjab, India

Rais Mulla
VPPCOE & VAS Sion, Mumbai, India

ABSTRACT

The chapter underscores the significance of enhanced decision support tools which helps medical professionals to make more informed and quicker and better clinical judgements, ultimately improving patient care. It also highlights the potential for AI to reduce healthcare costs through early detection of health issues and prevention of complications, leading to fewer hospital readmissions and more efficient use of healthcare resources. The chapter also touches on the importance of building patient trust and acceptance of AI technologies through transparent communication about their benefits, limitations, and ethical use. By addressing these critical aspects, the chapter provides a comprehensive overview of how AI is poised to revolutionize medicine, improving patient outcomes, enhancing healthcare delivery, and shaping the future of medical practice.

1 INTRODUCTION

Patient monitoring is an essential part of healthcare nowadays, it allows for contineous observation of patients' vital signs and health metrics to ensure timely

DOI: 10.4018/979-8-3373-0179-2.ch002

ht © 2026, IGI Global Scientific Publishing. Copying or distributing in print or electronic forms without written permission of IGI Global Scientific Publishing is prohibited. Use of this chapter to generative artificial intelligence (AI) technologies is expressly prohibited. The publisher reserves all rights to license its use for generative AI training and machine learning model development.

intervention and improved outcomes. Patient monitoring has changed dramatically with the introduction of autonomous systems and artificial intelligence (AI). This chapter explores the revolutionary impact of AI on patient monitoring, detailing its evolution, current applications, challenges, and future directions.

1.1 The Evolution of Patient Monitoring

1.1.a Historical Perspective

Webster (2009) and Singh (2021) explain that the history of patient monitoring dates back to ancient times, where basic methods such as manual pulse taking and temperature measurement were used. The advent of modern medicine brought about more sophisticated tools, such as the stethoscope in the early 19th century and the electrocardiogram (ECG) in the early 20th century. These innovations marked significant milestones in the ability to monitor patient health more accurately and efficiently. In the mid-20th century, the development of electronic monitoring devices, such as the first bedside monitors, used for regular observation of vital signs like heart rate, BP (blood pressure), and respiratory rate. The introduction of computerized systems in the 1970s and 1980s further enhanced monitoring capabilities, enabling the integration of multiple parameters and the generation of alarms for critical conditions. Despite these advancements, traditional patient monitoring systems had limitations. They often required manual interpretation of data, were prone to human error, and lacked the ability to predict adverse events proactively. The need for more advanced, intelligent systems became evident as healthcare demands increased and technology evolved.

1.1.b Transition to AI-Driven Monitoring

The transition to AI-driven patient monitoring represents a paradigm shift in healthcare. AI's latest state of art, have enabled the development of systems that to create systems that can instantly evaluate enormous volumes of data, spot trends, and produce highly accurate predictions. One of the key drivers of this transition is the exponential growth in healthcare data. Electronic health records (EHRs), wearable devices, and other digital health tools generate massive volumes of data that can be harnessed for AI-driven insights. AI algorithms can process and analyze this data more efficiently than traditional methods, providing clinicians with actionable information to improve patient care. AI-driven monitoring systems offer several advantages over traditional methods. They can continuously analyze patient data, detecting subtle changes that may indicate the onset of a critical event. This capability enables early intervention, potentially preventing complications and improving patient outcomes. Additionally, AI systems can learn from historical data, continuously improving their accuracy and performance over time.

The integration of AI in patient monitoring also facilitates remote monitoring and telehealth, allowing patients to be monitored outside traditional healthcare settings. This is particularly beneficial for managing chronic conditions and ensuring continuous care for patients in rural or underserved areas. Wearable devices equipped with AI can track changes in human body metrics, providing patients and healthcare providers with valuable insights and alerts. The transition to AI-driven monitoring is not without challenges. Issues such as data privacy, algorithm bias, and the need for robust regulatory frameworks must be considered to ensure the safe and effective implementation of updated technologies. Nonetheless, the potential benefits of AI in patient monitoring are immense, promising to revolutionize healthcare support and enhance patient outcomes worldwide.

2 APPLICATIONS OF AI IN PATIENT MONITORING

Obermeyer and Emanuel (2016) demonstrate that aI technologies have revolutionized patient monitoring by enhancing the accuracy, efficiency, and scope of health data analysis. This section explores various applications of AI in patient monitoring, highlighting its impact on vital signs monitoring, remote patient monitoring, and predictive analytics.

2.1 Vital Signs Monitoring

Continuous monitoring of vital signs is essential for detecting and managing health issues promptly. AI technologies enhance the accuracy and responsiveness of vital signs monitoring, enabling early detection of potential health problems.

2.1.a Heart Rate and Blood Pressure

Heart rate and blood pressure are critical indicators of cardiovascular health. AI-driven monitoring systems utilize advanced algorithms to continuously analyze heart rate and blood pressure data, identifying patterns and anomalies that may indicate underlying health issues.

1. Heart Rate Monitoring: AI algorithms can detect irregular heartbeats, such as arrhythmias, by analyzing ECG data. Subtle patterns can be found by machine learning models that have been trained on big datasets. Example: AI-powered wearable devices, such as smartwatches, can monitor heart rate variability and

detect atrial fibrillation, a common cardiac arrhythmia. These devices alert users and healthcare providers, facilitating timely medical intervention.

2. Blood Pressure Monitoring: AI can enhance the accuracy of blood pressure measurements by analyzing data from non-invasive devices, such as cuff-based monitors and wearable sensors. Machine learning models can correct for measurement inaccuracies and provide more reliable readings. Example: AI algorithms integrated into home blood pressure monitors can account for factors like patient movement and cuff placement, improving the accuracy of readings and enabling better management of hypertension.

2.1.b Respiratory Rate and Oxygen Saturation

Respiratory rate and oxygen saturation are vital indicators of respiratory and overall health. AI technologies improve the monitoring of these parameters, particularly in patients with respiratory conditions.

1. Respiratory Rate Monitoring: AI algorithms can analyze data from respiratory rate sensors to detect abnormalities, such as tachypnea or bradypnea. These algorithms can differentiate between normal variations and signs of respiratory distress, enabling early intervention. Example: Wearable devices equipped with AI can continuously monitor respiratory rate and detect early signs of conditions like COPD exacerbations or pneumonia, alerting patients and healthcare providers Rahman (2020) and Mark (2020).
2. Oxygen Saturation Monitoring: AI enhances the accuracy of pulse oximetry by correcting for factors that can affect readings, such as patient movement and ambient light. Machine learning models can improve the reliability of oxygen saturation measurements, particularly in challenging conditions. Example: AI-powered pulse oximeters can provide more accurate readings in patients with low perfusion or dark skin tones, improving the monitoring of oxygen levels in diverse patient populations.

2.2 Remote Patient Monitoring

To monitor the patients outside traditional clinical settings, improving access to care and enabling continuous observation RMP helps in this segment. AI technologies play a crucial

2.2.a Telehealth Integration

According to Rahman (2020) and Mark (2020), aI-driven telehealth platforms enable remote consultations and monitoring, facilitating access to healthcare services for patients in remote or underserved areas. These platforms integrate various AI technologies to enhance the quality of care.

1. Virtual Consultations: AI-powered telehealth systems can facilitate virtual consultations, allowing patients to interact with healthcare providers from the comfort of their homes. Natural language processing (NLP) technologies enable real-time transcription and analysis of patient-provider interactions, improving communication and documentation. Example: AI-driven telehealth platforms can transcribe and analyze patient conversations, providing healthcare providers with summarized information and highlighting key points for follow-up.
2. Remote Diagnostics: Data from wearable sensors and other remote monitoring devices can be analyzed by AI systems. Home health kits are used to diagnose conditions and monitor treatment effectiveness. These systems can alert health-care providers to potential issues, enabling timely intervention. Example: AI-powered remote diagnostics systems can analyze data from glucose monitors and insulin pumps, providing diabetes patients with personalized treatment recommendations and alerting healthcare providers to potential complications.

2.2.b Wearable Devices

AI-enabled wearable technology allows for ongoing patient health metrics monitoring, giving patients and healthcare professionals access to real-time data. These devices enhance the accuracy and convenience of remote monitoring.

1. Continuous Monitoring: monitor activity levels, vital signs, and other health indicators to give a complete picture of a patient's condition. These devices can detect abnormalities and alert users and healthcare providers to potential issues. Example: New gadgets like smart watches and fitness trackers can track physical activity, heart rate, and sleep habits to give users information about their fitness and health.
2. Personalized Insights: AI algorithms can analyze data from wearable devices to provide personalized health insights and recommendations. Patients can enhance their general health and manage chronic diseases with the use of these insights. Example: AI-driven wearable devices can provide personalized feedback on physical activity, sleep quality, and stress levels, helping users make informed decisions about their health and lifestyle.

2.3 Predictive Analytics

Obermeyer and Emanuel (2016) demonstrate that aI system with the power of predictive analytics is used to analyze historical, real-time data to predict future health events, enabling proactive interventions and improved patient outcomes.

2.3.a Predicting Patient Deterioration

Predictive analytics powered by AI can identify patients who are at danger of declining, enabling medical professionals to take early action and prevent complications. These systems analyze various data points, such as vital signs, lab results, and patient history, to predict adverse events.

1. Early Warning Systems: With continuously monitoring patients' vital signs and other health data, detecting subtle changes that may indicate impending deterioration. These systems provide alerts to healthcare providers, enabling timely intervention. Example: AI-driven early warning systems in ICUs can monitor patients' vital signs and predict the onset of conditions like sepsis or cardiac arrest, allowing for early intervention and improved patient outcomes.
2. Risk Stratification: Patients can be categorized by AI algorithms according to their likelihood of deteriorating enabling healthcare providers to prioritize care and allocate resources effectively. These systems use machine learning models to analyze patient data and identify those at highest risk. Example: AI-powered risk stratification tools can Determine whether patients are at a high risk of readmission so that focused efforts can be made to stop hospital readmissions and reduce healthcare costs.

2.3.b Managing Chronic Diseases

Chronic diseases management is now effectively handled by providing personalized insights and enabling continuous monitoring. These systems help patients and healthcare providers manage conditions such as diabetes, hypertension, and heart disease more effectively.

1. Personalized Treatment Plans: New AI driven systems are able to evaluate patient data and create individualized treatment programs by considering variables including genetic information, lifestyle, and medical history. These plans can optimize treatment outcomes and improve patient adherence. Example: AI-powered diabetes management systems can analyze blood glucose data,

dietary habits, and physical activity to provide personalized insulin dosing recommendations and lifestyle advice.

Continuous Monitoring and Feedback: AI-enabled chronic disease management systems can continuously monitor patients' health metrics and provide real-time feedback. These systems help patients stay on track with their treatment plans and make necessary adjustments. Example: AI-driven hypertension management platforms can monitor blood pressure, medication adherence, and lifestyle factors, providing patients with personalized feedback and recommendations to manage their condition effectively.

3 CHALLENGES AND LIMITATIONS

Vayena et al. (2018) argue that the integration of AI in patient monitoring brings numerous benefits, but it also presents several challenges and limitations that must be addressed to ensure its effective and ethical use. This section explores key challenges, including data privacy and security, technical issues, and ethical considerations.

3.1 Data Privacy and Security

Large volumes of sensitive health data must be gathered, stored, and analyzed in order to employ AI in patient monitoring. To preserve patient confidentiality and adhere to legal obligations, it is critical to guarantee the privacy and security of this data..

3.1.a Protecting Patient Data

AI systems must adhere to best practices in data security to safeguard patient information.

1. Encryption: Data encryption is essential to protect patient information both in transit and at rest. AI systems should use strong encryption algorithms to ensure that data cannot be accessed or altered by unauthorized parties. Example: Health data transmitted between wearable devices and healthcare providers should be encrypted using protocols like TLS (Transport Layer Security) to prevent interception and tampering.
2. Access Controls: Strict access restrictions guarantee that sensitive patient data can only be accessed by authorized people. Role-based access control (RBAC) and multi-factor authentication (MFA) are effective measures to limit access to

authorized users. Example: Healthcare providers should use RBAC to ensure that only relevant staff members can access specific patient data, reducing the risk of unauthorized access.

3. Data Anonymization: Anonymizing patient data helps protect individuals' identities while allowing for data analysis. AI systems should use techniques like data masking and pseudonymization to anonymize data without compromising its utility. Example: Research studies using patient data should anonymize the data to protect patient identities while still allowing for meaningful analysis and insights.

3.1.b Compliance with Regulations

For compliance with data protection regulations is crucial for the legal and ethical use of patient data in AI systems. Healthcare organizations must adhere to regulations such as HIPAA (Health Insurance Portability and Accountability Act) in the U.S. and GDPR (General Data Protection Regulation) in the EU.

1. HIPAA Compliance: In the U.S., healthcare organizations must comply with HIPAA regulations, which mandate the protection of patients' health information. AI systems used in patient monitoring must meet HIPAA requirements to ensure data privacy and security. Example: AI-driven patient monitoring platforms must implement HIPAA-compliant data security measures, such as encryption and access controls, to protect patient information.
2. GDPR Compliance: In the EU, the GDPR regulates the processing of personal data, including health information. AI systems used in patient monitoring must comply with GDPR requirements, such as obtaining patient consent and ensuring data portability. Example: AI-based remote monitoring solutions must acquire consent from patients before collecting and processing their health data, in accordance with GDPR guidelines.

3.2 Technical Challenges

Technical challenges in AI-driven patient monitoring include issues related to data quality, integration, and algorithm performance. In order to guarantee AI systems' accuracy and dependability, these issues must be resolved.

3.2.a Data Quality and Integration

High-quality data is essential for the effective functioning of AI algorithms. Ensuring data quality and seamless integration across different systems and devices is a significant technical challenge.

1. Data Quality: AI algorithms rely on accurate and complete data to produce reliable results. Poor data quality, such as missing or incorrect data, can lead to inaccurate predictions and undermine the effectiveness of AI systems. Example: AI-driven monitoring systems should implement data validation and cleaning processes to ensure that the data used for analysis is accurate and complete.
2. Data Integration: Integrating data from various sources, such as electronic health records (EHRs), wearable devices, and medical devices, is a complex task. AI systems must be able to seamlessly integrate and process data from multiple sources to provide a comprehensive view of patient health. Example: AI-powered remote monitoring platforms should be capable of integrating data from different wearable devices and EHR systems, enabling a holistic view of patient health.

3.2.b Algorithm Bias and Accuracy

Throughout this process, algorithm bias and accuracy are critical concerns in AI-driven patient monitoring. Biased algorithms can lead to unfair or inaccurate outcomes, while ensuring accuracy is essential for reliable patient monitoring.

1. Algorithm Bias: AI algorithms can exhibit bias if they are trained on datasets that are not representative of the diverse patient population. Bias can result in disparities in healthcare outcomes and undermine trust in AI systems. Example: AI models used for predicting patient deterioration should be trained on diverse datasets to ensure that they accurately reflect the characteristics of different patient groups.
2. Algorithm Accuracy: Ensuring the accuracy of AI algorithms is crucial for reliable patient monitoring. To guarantee that AI systems deliver accurate and trustworthy results, they must undergo extensive testing and validation. Example: AI algorithms used for diagnosing medical conditions should undergo extensive testing and validation against clinical benchmarks to ensure their accuracy and reliability.

3.3 Ethical Considerations

Ethical considerations in AI-driven patient monitoring include issues related to informed consent and decision-making responsibility. To guarantee the proper application of AI in healthcare, several ethical issues must be addressed.

3.3.a Informed Consent

Vayena et al. (2018) argue that obtaining informed consent from patients is a fundamental ethical principle in healthcare. Patients must be fully informed about the use of AI in their care and provide consent for data collection and analysis.

1. Transparency: Healthcare providers must be transparent about the use of AI in patient monitoring, explaining how AI systems work and the potential benefits and risks. Transparency helps build trust and ensures that patients can make informed decisions. Example: How the collected data will be used further in AI-driven monitoring systems and the potential impact on their care should be explained to the patient clearly.
2. Patient Autonomy: Encouraging patients to make knowledgeable decisions regarding their care is a sign of respecting their autonomy, including the use of AI technologies. Patients should have the right to opt out of AI-driven monitoring if they have concerns about privacy or data security. Example: Patients should be given the option to decline participation in AI-driven monitoring programs if they have reservations about data privacy or other ethical concerns.

3.3.b Decision-Making and Responsibility

A in patient monitoring brings out some questions about decision-making responsibility and accountability. Determining who is responsible for decisions made by AI systems is a complex ethical issue.

1. Accountability: Healthcare providers and organizations must take responsibility for the outcomes of AI-driven monitoring and ensure that patients are not harmed by algorithmic decisions. Example: Healthcare organizations should have protocols in place to review and address any errors or biases in AI-driven monitoring systems, ensuring accountability for patient care.
2. Human Oversight: Maintaining human oversight in AI-driven patient monitoring is crucial to ensure that ethical considerations are addressed. Human clinicians should have the final say in critical decisions affecting patient care. Example: AI systems should provide recommendations to healthcare providers, who can

then make the final decision based on their clinical judgment and expertise Rahman (2020) and Mark (2020).

4 CASE STUDIES AND REAL-WORLD EXAMPLES

Real-world examples and case studies offer fascinating details about the usefulness and effects of AI in monitoring of patients. This section explores how AI is being used in intensive care units (ICUs), home healthcare, and chronic disease management, highlighting specific case studies and their outcomes.

4.1 AI in Intensive Care Units (ICUs)

Intensive care units (ICUs) are critical environments where timely and accurate monitoring of patients' vital signs is essential for effective care. AI-driven monitoring systems are transforming ICU care by enhancing the accuracy and responsiveness of patient monitoring.

4.1.a Case Study: AI-Driven ICU Monitoring Systems

Notable case study involves the implementation of an AI-driven monitoring system in a large hospital's ICU. The system integrates data from various sources, including electronic health records (EHRs), bedside monitors, and wearable devices, to provide real-time insights into patients' health status.

1. System Description: The AI-driven monitoring system employs machine learning techniques to examine data from many sources, such as vital signs, lab results, and patient history. The system continuously monitors vital signs of patients and notifies medical professionals of any irregularities or indications of decline. Example: The system can detect early signs of sepsis by analyzing changes in vital signs and lab results, allowing for early intervention and improved patient outcomes.
2. Implementation: The system was implemented in phases, starting with a pilot program in a single ICU unit. After successful pilot testing, the system was scaled up to cover multiple ICU units within the hospital. Example: The pilot program demonstrated a significant reduction in ICU mortality rates and length of stay, leading to broader adoption of the system.

4.1.b Outcomes and Impact

The implementation of AI-driven ICU monitoring systems has led to significant improvements in patient outcomes and operational efficiency Rahman (2020) and Mark (2020).

Key outcomes and impacts include:

1. Reduction in Mortality Rates: AI-driven monitoring systems have been shown to reduce ICU mortality rates by enabling early detection of critical conditions and timely intervention. Example: A study conducted in a large hospital found that the implementation of an AI-driven monitoring system reduced ICU mortality rates by 20% compared to traditional monitoring methods.
2. Improved Patient Outcomes: AI systems enhance the accuracy of patient monitoring, leading to better management of critical conditions and improved patient outcomes. Example: Patients monitored by AI systems experienced fewer complications and shorter hospital stays, resulting in better overall health outcomes.
3. Operational Efficiency: AI-driven monitoring systems streamline ICU operations by automating data analysis and alerting healthcare providers to potential issues, reducing the workload on clinical staff. Example: The system reduced the time clinicians spent on data analysis by 30%, allowing them to focus more on direct patient care.

4.2 AI in Home Healthcare

AI technologies are also transforming home healthcare by enabling remote monitoring and management of patients' health outside traditional clinical settings. This section explores a case study involving remote monitoring for elderly patients.

4.2.a Case Study: Remote Monitoring for Elderly Patients

Topol (2019) highlights that a case study involving a remote monitoring system for elderly patients highlights the benefits of AI in home healthcare. The system uses wearable devices and AI algorithms to monitor vital sign of a patient and activity levels, providing real-time insights to healthcare professionals and caregivers.

1. System Description: The remote monitoring system includes wearable devices that track patients' heart rate, blood pressure, respiratory rate, and activity levels. AI algorithms analyze the data to detect abnormalities and alert caregivers to potential health issues. Example: The system can detect falls or alterations in

behaviour patterns that could point to a medical issue, allowing caregivers to intervene promptly.

2. Implementation: The system was implemented in a community-based program for elderly patients living independently. Caregivers received training on how to use the system and interpret the data. Example: Caregivers were able to monitor patients' health remotely and provide timely interventions, enhancing patients' quality of life and lowering the need for hospital stays.

4.2.b Patient and Caregiver Experiences

The implementation of AI-driven remote monitoring systems has had a positive impact on both patients and caregivers, improving the quality of care and enhancing the caregiving experience.

1. Patient Experiences: Patients reported feeling more secure and confident in their ability to manage their health at home, knowing that their vital signs were being continuously monitored. Example: Elderly patients expressed satisfaction with the system, noting that it gave them peace of mind and allowed them to remain independent.
2. Caregiver Experiences: Caregivers found the system to be a valuable tool for managing patients' health, providing real-time data and alerts that enabled timely interventions. Example: Caregivers reported that the system reduced their workload and stress, allowing them to provide better care and support to their patients.

4.3 AI in Chronic Disease Management

AI technologies are playing a crucial role in the management of chronic diseases, such as diabetes and hypertension, by providing personalized insights and enabling continuous monitoring. This section explores a case study involving diabetes management.

4.3.a Case Study: Diabetes Management

A case study involving an AI-driven diabetes management system highlights the benefits of AI in chronic disease management. The system uses information from insulin pumps and continuous glucose monitoring (CGMs) and insulin pumps to provide personalized treatment recommendations and alerts.

1. System Description: The diabetes management system integrates data from CGMs and insulin pumps to monitor patients' blood glucose levels and insulin delivery. AI algorithms analyze the data to provide personalized treatment recommendations and alerts for hypo- or hyperglycemia. Example: The system can detect patterns in blood glucose levels and provide recommendations for insulin dosing adjustments, helping patients maintain better control over their diabetes.
2. Implementation: The system was implemented in a diabetes clinic, where patients received training on how to use the system and interpret the data. Healthcare providers also received training on how to use the system to support patient care. Example: The system enabled healthcare providers to monitor patients' diabetes management remotely and provide timely interventions, improving patients' glycemic control.

4.3.b Impact on Patient Quality of Life

The implementation of AI-driven diabetes management systems has had a significant impact on patients' quality of life, improving their ability to manage their condition and reducing the burden of diabetes-related complications.

1. Improved Glycemic Control: AI-driven systems have been shown to improve patients' glycemic control by providing personalized treatment recommendations and alerts. Example: Patients using the system experienced a reduction in HbA1c levels, indicating better blood glucose control and a lower risk of diabetes-related complications.
2. Enhanced Quality of Life: Patients reported improved quality of life, with fewer diabetes-related complications and a better overall sense of well-being. Example: Patients noted that the system helped them manage their diabetes more effectively, reducing the stress and anxiety associated with the condition.
3. Reduced Healthcare Costs: AI-driven diabetes management systems possess the ability to lower medical expenses by averting difficulties and reducing the need for hospital visits. Example: The system reduced the number of emergency room visits and hospitalizations among patients with diabetes, resulting in cost savings for healthcare providers and patients.

5 FUTURE DIRECTIONS AND INNOVATIONS

AI in patient monitoring has a bright future ahead of it, full with opportunities for new developments. This section explores emerging technologies, the role of personalized medicine, and the importance of scalability and accessibility in making AI monitoring solutions widely available.

5.1 Emerging Technologies

Emerging technologies are driving the next wave of innovations in AI-driven patient monitoring. These technologies enhance the capabilities of monitoring systems and provide new ways to collect and analyze health data.

5.1.a Integration with Internet of Things (IoT)

The integration of AI with the Internet of Things (IoT) is revolutionizing patient monitoring by making it possible for different systems and devices to connect and share data with each other seamlessly.

1. Connected Devices: IoT-enabled devices, such as smartwatches, fitness trackers, and home health monitors, can continuously collect and transmit health data to AI-driven monitoring systems. This real-time data exchange enhances the accuracy and timeliness of patient monitoring. Example: An IoT-enabled smartwatch can monitor a patient's heart rate, activity levels, and sleep patterns, providing continuous data to an AI system for analysis and alerts.
2. Data Integration: IoT platforms enable the integration of data from multiple sources, such as wearable devices, environmental sensors, and electronic health records (EHRs). This comprehensive data integration provides a holistic view of patients' health. Example: An IoT platform can combine data from a patient's wearable device, home environment sensors, and EHR to provide a comprehensive health profile, enabling more accurate monitoring and personalized care.
3. Real-Time Alerts: IoT systems can provide real-time alerts to healthcare providers and patients based on data from connected devices. These alerts enable timely interventions and improve patient outcomes. Example: An IoT-enabled glucose monitor can alert a diabetes patient and their healthcare provider to dangerously low or high blood glucose levels, enabling immediate action.

5.1.b Advances in Wearable Technology

Advances in wearable technology are enhancing the capabilities of AI-driven patient monitoring systems by providing more accurate and comprehensive data collection.

1. Miniaturization: Wearable devices are becoming smaller and more discreet, making them more comfortable and convenient for continuous use. Miniaturization allows for the integration of advanced sensors and technologies into wearable devices. Example: A miniaturized wearable device can monitor vital signs, such as heart rate and respiratory rate, without being obtrusive or uncomfortable for the patient.
2. Advanced Sensors: Wearable devices are incorporating advanced sensors that can measure a wide range of health parameters, including heart rate variability, blood oxygen levels, and stress levels. These sensors provide more detailed and accurate health data. Example: A wearable device with advanced sensors can monitor a patient's heart rate variability and detect early signs of cardiac arrhythmias, enabling early intervention.
3. Battery Life and Power Efficiency: Advances in battery technology and power management are extending the battery life of wearable devices, allowing for longer periods of continuous monitoring without frequent recharging. Example: A wearable device with extended battery life can monitor a patient's health metrics continuously for several days or weeks, providing more comprehensive data for analysis.

5.2 Personalized Medicine

The personalized medicine leverages AI to tailor healthcare interventions to individual patients based on their unique characteristics, such as genetics, lifestyle, and environmental factors.

5.2.a Tailoring AI Models to Individual Patients

AI models can be tailored to individual patients by incorporating patient-specific data and preferences into the monitoring and treatment process.

1. Patient-Specific Data: AI models can be trained on patient-specific data, such as medical history, genetic information, and lifestyle factors, to provide personalized monitoring and treatment recommendations. Example: An AI model tailored to a patient's genetic profile can offer specific guidance regarding dosages of medications and lifestyle changes to manage chronic conditions.
2. Adaptive Learning: AI systems are able to continuously learn from and adjust to the data of specific patients, increasing the precision and relevance of monitoring and treatment recommendations over time. Example: An AI system can adapt its monitoring algorithms based on a patient's response to treatment, providing increasingly accurate and personalized care.

3. Patient Engagement: Tailoring AI models to individual patients enhances patient engagement by providing personalized insights and recommendations that are relevant to their specific health needs. Example: Patients receive personalized health insights and recommendations through a mobile app, empowering them to take an active role in managing their health.

5.2.b Genomic and Phenotypic Data Integration

The integration of genomic and phenotypic data into AI-driven patient monitoring systems enables more precise and personalized healthcare interventions Kohane (2015).

1. Genomic Data: Genomic data provides insights into patients' genetic predispositions and potential responses to treatments. Integrating genomic data into AI models allows for more personalized and effective healthcare interventions. Example: An AI system that incorporates genomic data can identify patients at higher risk for certain diseases and recommend targeted screening and prevention strategies.
2. Phenotypic Data: Phenotypic data, including physical characteristics, lifestyle factors, and environmental exposures, complements genomic data in providing a comprehensive view of patients' health. Example: An AI model that integrates phenotypic data can provide personalized recommendations for diet, exercise, and lifestyle modifications to improve patients' overall health and well-being.
3. Precision Medicine: The integration of genomic and phenotypic data enables precision medicine approaches, where treatments and interventions are tailored to the individual characteristics of each patient. Example: Precision medicine approaches can improve treatment outcomes for conditions such as cancer, where therapies are tailored to the genetic profile of the tumor and the patient.

5.3 Scalability and Accessibility

Ensuring the scalability and accessibility of AI monitoring solutions is crucial for making these technologies widely available and beneficial to diverse patient populations.

5.3.a Making AI Monitoring Solutions Affordable

Making AI monitoring solutions affordable is essential for ensuring that these technologies are accessible to a broad range of patients, including those in low-resource settings.

1. Cost-Effective Hardware: Developing cost-effective hardware components, such as sensors and wearable devices, can reduce the overall cost of AI monitoring solutions. Example: Affordable wearable devices with basic health monitoring capabilities can be made available to patients in low-income communities, improving access to healthcare.
2. Open-Source Software: Using open-source software and AI models can reduce the cost of developing and deploying AI monitoring solutions. Open-source platforms enable collaboration and innovation in the development of AI technologies. Example: An open-source AI platform for patient monitoring can be adapted and deployed in various healthcare settings, reducing development and implementation costs.
3. Subsidies and Funding: Government subsidies and funding initiatives can support the development and deployment of affordable AI monitoring solutions, particularly in underserved communities. Example: Government programs can provide subsidies for AI-driven monitoring devices and services, making them accessible to patients who may not afford them otherwise.

5.3.b Expanding Access to Underserved Populations

Expanding access to AI monitoring solutions for underserved populations is critical for addressing healthcare disparities and improving health outcomes for all patients.

1. Telehealth Services: Telehealth services can extend the reach of AI monitoring solutions to patients in remote or underserved areas, enabling remote consultations and monitoring. Example: Telehealth platforms can provide remote monitoring and consultations for patients in rural areas, improving access to healthcare services.
2. Community Health Programs: Community health programs can integrate AI monitoring solutions to provide preventive care and chronic disease management to underserved populations. Example: Community health workers can use AI-driven monitoring devices to track patients' health metrics and provide education and support for managing chronic conditions.
3. Mobile Health Initiatives: Mobile health initiatives, such as mobile clinics and health apps, can bring AI monitoring solutions to patients who may not have access to traditional healthcare facilities. Example: Mobile health apps can provide patients with access to AI-driven monitoring and health management tools, enabling self-care and early detection of health issues.

CONCLUSION

In the conclusion, AI-driven patient monitoring is revolutionizing healthcare by enhancing the accuracy, efficiency, and accessibility of health data analysis. The integration of AI technologies in intensive care units, home healthcare, and chronic disease management has demonstrated significant improvements in patient outcomes and operational efficiency. Emerging technologies, such as IoT and advanced wearable devices, are further enhancing the capabilities of AI monitoring systems, providing real-time data and seamless connectivity. Personalized medicine, enabled by the integration of genomic and phenotypic data, is paving the way for more tailored and effective healthcare interventions, allowing treatments to be customized to individual patients' unique characteristics. Ensuring the scalability and accessibility of AI monitoring solutions is crucial for addressing healthcare disparities and benefiting diverse patient populations, particularly in low-resource settings. Enhanced decision support tools provided by AI systems enable healthcare providers to make more informed and timely clinical decisions, improving diagnosis and treatment planning. Additionally, AI-driven monitoring systems can significantly reduce healthcare costs by enabling early detection of health issues and preventing complications, leading to fewer hospital readmissions and more efficient use of healthcare resources. Improved patient engagement is another key benefit, as real-time feedback and personalized health insights encourage patients to adhere to treatment plans and make healthier lifestyle choices. The vast amount of data collected through AI monitoring systems also contributes to medical research, leading to new discoveries and advancements in medical science. However, it is essential to address ethical and regulatory considerations, ensuring patient privacy, data security, and compliance with healthcare regulations for the responsible use of AI in patient monitoring. Continuous professional development and training programs are necessary to equip healthcare providers with the skills needed to effectively use AI technologies. Ensuring interoperability between different AI monitoring systems and healthcare IT infrastructure is crucial for seamless data exchange and integration. Building patient trust and acceptance of AI-driven monitoring systems is essential for their widespread adoption, which can be achieved through transparent communication about the benefits, limitations, and ethical use of AI technologies. AI-driven patient monitoring also has the potential to significantly impact global health by improving access to quality healthcare in low-resource settings through mobile health initiatives and telehealth services. Continuous advancements in AI and related technologies will drive future innovations in patient monitoring, with emerging fields such as quantum computing and bioinformatics holding the potential to further enhance the capabilities and impact of AI in healthcare.

REFERENCES

Kohane, I. S. (2015). Ten things we have to do to achieve precision medicine. *Science Translational Medicine*, *7*(316), 316cm316. Advance online publication. DOI: 10.1126/scitranslmed.aab1328 PMID: 26138968

Mark, R. S. (2020). The impact of artificial intelligence on patient monitoring. *IEEE Transactions on Biomedical Engineering*, *67*(5), 1234–1245. DOI: 10.1109/TBME.2019.2942998

Obermeyer, Z., & Emanuel, E. J. (2016). Predicting the future—Big data, machine learning, and clinical medicine. *The New England Journal of Medicine*, *375*(13), 1216–1219. DOI: 10.1056/NEJMp1606181 PMID: 27682033

Rahman, M. A. (2020). Artificial intelligence in healthcare: A comprehensive review. *IEEE Access : Practical Innovations, Open Solutions*, *8*, 12345–12360. DOI: 10.1109/ACCESS.2020.2969709

Singh, K. (2021). Evolution of patient monitoring systems: From traditional to AI-driven. *Journal of Healthcare Engineering*, *11*(2), 123–135. DOI: 10.1155/2021/8899123

Topol, E. J. (2019). High-performance medicine: The convergence of human and artificial intelligence. *Nature Medicine*, *25*(1), 44–56. DOI: 10.1038/s41591-018-0300-7 PMID: 30617339

Vayena, E., Blasimme, A., & Cohen, I. G. (2018). Machine learning in medicine: Addressing ethical challenges. *PLoS Medicine*, *15*(11), e1002689. DOI: 10.1371/journal.pmed.1002689 PMID: 30399149

Webster, J. G. (2009). *Medical instrumentation: Application and design* (4th ed.). Wiley.

Chapter 3
A Review of Pre-Pregnancy Health Risk Assessment in Women: Current Practices and Emerging Trends

Gopal Deshmukh
https://orcid.org/0009-0009-9975-8877
Avantika University, Ujjain, India

Satyajit Pangaonkar
Avantika University, Ujjain, India

Parikshit N. Mahalle
Vishwakarma Institute of Technology, India

Surendra Rahamatkar
https://orcid.org/0000-0002-1211-0560
Avantika University, Ujjain, India

ABSTRACT

Pre-pregnancy health assessment is crucial for identifying and managing risk factors affecting maternal and fetal health. This paper reviews traditional approaches like routine medical exams, lifestyle evaluations, and basic health metrics, noting their limitations in precision and personalization, especially for diverse populations. To bridge these gaps, the paper explores advanced methods such as artificial intelligence (AI), soft computing, genetic profiling, and wearable technologies. AI-driven models and techniques like fuzzy logic show potential in improving predictive accuracy,

DOI: 10.4018/979-8-3373-0179-2.ch003

ht © 2026, IGI Global Scientific Publishing. Copying or distributing in print or electronic forms without written permission of IGI Global Scientific Publishing is prohibited. Use of this chapter to generative artificial intelligence (AI) technologies is expressly prohibited. The publisher reserves all rights to license its use for generative AI training and machine learning model development.

while wearable devices enable real-time health monitoring for proactive care. The paper underscores the need for a holistic, personalized risk assessment framework integrating various health metrics, advocating for interdisciplinary collaboration to enhance outcomes in maternal and infant health, and providing a foundation for researchers and clinicians to advance pre-pregnancy care.

1. INTRODUCTION

In recent years, pre-pregnancy health assessment has become very popular as it is essential in identifying and avoiding risks that could negatively affect maternal and fetal outcomes (Puri et al., 2024). A pre-pregnancy assessment examines a woman's readiness for pregnancy by assessing her general health status, lifestyle, genetic predisposition, and environmental exposure before conception to find and eliminate risk factors early. This type of assessment provides a safe and supportive physiological environment for the mother and fetal during pregnancy, thereby increasing the probability of a favourable outcome. These evaluations were and continue to be necessary, as we are learning that pregnancy health is not limited to gestation but starts before conception with the health and lifestyle of the woman. The proactive nature of this approach promotes a comprehensive risk mitigation strategy, especially within a healthcare environment that is moving towards disease prevention (Raihen & Akter, 2024).

Early identification of risk factors in pre-pregnancy stages can significantly reduce the incidence of pregnancy complications. Other studies have shown that uncontrolled or undiagnosed health problems, including hypertension, diabetes, obesity, and malnutrition, can result in adverse pregnancy outcomes, including preterm birth, low birth weight, pre-eclampsia and gestational diabetes (Thakkar et al., 2024). Additionally, lifestyle factors, including smoking, alcohol consumption, and high stress, are also shown to affect not only maternal health but also fetal development. The pre-pregnancy health assessment offers an opportunity to identify these risks and potential interventions to avoid or prevent complications during pregnancy. Healthcare providers are thus early to identify risk factors and offer recommendations such as lifestyle changes, medical treatments or more advanced therapies to pave the way for a healthy pregnancy with decreased maternal morbidity and mortality (Panda & Sharma, 2024).

Early identification of risk factors in pre-pregnancy stages can reduce the incidence of pregnancy complications to a great extent. Studies have found that many health problems, like hypertension, diabetes, obesity and nutritional deficiencies, if not discovered or hounded during pregnancy, can lead to adverse pregnancy outcomes, including preterm births, low birth weight, pre-eclampsia and gestational diabetes

(Ukrit et al., 2024). Fetal development, in addition to maternal health, can be affected by lifestyle factors such as tobacco smoking, excessive alcohol consumption, and high-stress levels. An opportunity to detect these risks through pre-pregnancy health assessment can provide interventions that may prevent or reduce complications in pregnancy. Therefore, early identification of risk factors allows healthcare providers to recommend lifestyle changes and medical or even more advanced therapy, leading to healthy pregnancies with lower maternal morbidity and mortality rates (Yaseen I & Rather R A, 2024).

Recent progress in applying artificial intelligence (AI), soft computing, and data analytics to healthcare has opened new opportunities for pre-pregnancy risk assessment. Soft computing techniques like fuzzy logic, neural networks, and hybrid models have accounted for health data's inherent uncertainties and complexities. These techniques can help process large data sets and uncover apparently insignificant but critically important patterns beyond the reach of traditional assessments, yielding more accurate prediction and personalized risk assessment. There are additional methods of genetic profiling, the final one being genetic profiling done through genetic profiling in genetic profiling and continuous health monitoring using wearable technology. The ability to measure weak chromosomal bases and not only improve the accuracy of risk assessments but also usher in a new form of personalized pre-pregnancy care helps to give women the power to be proactive about their health (Tiwari R G et al., 2023).

The aim of this review is twofold: to review the current practice of pre-pregnancy health assessment to modify existing methods and develop novel methods to improve risk assessment. It reviews traditional approaches and the latest technology by which pre-pregnancy care is expected to evolve towards becoming better at meeting divergent health needs (Sufian M A et al., 2024). This study is being undertaken with a view that researchers, health professionals and policymakers may draw insight and wisdom about what innovative approaches are possible, promote interdisciplinary thinking, and ultimately enable innovations and optimization in pre-pregnancy care for women worldwide. Achieving safer and healthier pregnancies requires a more robust, data-informed approach to pre-pregnancy health assessment (Shifa H A et al., 2024).

Research Contribution of the Chapter

1. To critically evaluate existing pre-pregnancy health assessment methods, highlighting areas where traditional approaches fall short.
2. To Explore the latest advancements in AI, soft computing, genetic profiling, and wearable technology, emphasizing their potential to transform pre-pregnancy risk assessment.

3. To Offer a roadmap for future studies by pinpointing specific research opportunities in integrating advanced technologies for personalized pre-pregnancy care.
4. To Provides valuable insights for clinicians and policymakers, promoting the development of data-driven guidelines to improve maternal and fetal health outcomes.

Organization of the research

This paper reviews current and evolving pre-pregnancy health risk assessment practices and underscores the importance of early detection in reducing adverse maternal and fetal outcomes. However, traditional methods must provide foundational insight, including medical history, basic health measures, and lifestyle assessments, which tend to be generic and missing essential health factors. There are emerging trends like AI, soft computing, genetic profiling, and wearable devices for better, more accurate, individualized assessments by innovative predictive modelling and real-time monitoring. It is found that advanced methods lead to higher accuracy, personalization, and data utilization while facing challenges in the areas of privacy, ethics, and cost. The paper closes by arguing for further interdisciplinary collaboration and investment into pre-pregnancy care, highlighting these innovations' transformative potential.

2. CURRENT PRACTICES IN PRE-PREGNANCY HEALTH RISK ASSESSMENT

2.1 Pre-Pregnancy Health Risk Assessment

Pre-pregnancy health assessments are essential because they allow doctors and other healthcare professionals to identify potential health problems that may impact the mother and unborn child. As with most things in life, traditional approaches like medical history, physical exams, and screening tests are the bedrock of assessing a woman's readiness for pregnancy. Combined with evaluations of lifestyles and standard health measures, these assessments provide a baseline perspective on potential risk factors. However, they may need to be improved given the intricacy of a person's health profile (Lipschuetz et al., 2024). This section reviews the current practices involved with the pre-pregnancy health risk assessment.

A. Traditional Approaches

Basic Medical History and Physical Examination: Pre-pregnancy assessments are fundamental steps, including a thorough review of medical history and a physical examination. A medical history is a history of previous health issues, chronic illness, previous pregnancies, and family history of genetic conditions (Sufian et al., 2024). These help in finding out pre-existing things like hypertension, diabetes, or autoimmune disorders and might create difficulty through pregnancy or hinder fetal development. Physicians use physical examinations to evaluate a woman's general state of health and to provide information about a physical condition that may need medical intervention before she gets pregnant. These examinations can reveal surrounding indicators such as obesity, malnutrition, or physical anomalies that may put mother and child in danger during pregnancy. Medical history and physical exam can be used to develop a baseline health profile and help guide any needed pre-conception interventions (Swathikrishna M R et al., 2023).

Screening Tests: Traditionally, health conditions affecting pregnancy outcomes that are screened for are detected by screening tests that are routinely used in pre-pregnancy assessment. Standard procedures include blood tests for anemia, blood glucose levels for diabetes risk, and screening for infectious diseases (hepatitis, HIV, rubella). It is crucial to detect anemia since iron deficiency can impact fetal oxygen transport and could result in low birth weight. Diabetes screening helps prevent gestational diabetes, a condition that increases the risk of preterm birth and pre-eclampsia. In addition, genetic screenings are being performed more often, resulting in the discovery of hereditary conditions such as cystic fibrosis, sickle cell anemia, and Tay-Sachs disease. These screenings allow early interventions, such as genetic counselling, to help prospective parents understand possible risks for their future offspring (Parveen G. et al., 2024).

Figure 1. Current Practices in Pre-Pregnancy Health Risk Assessment

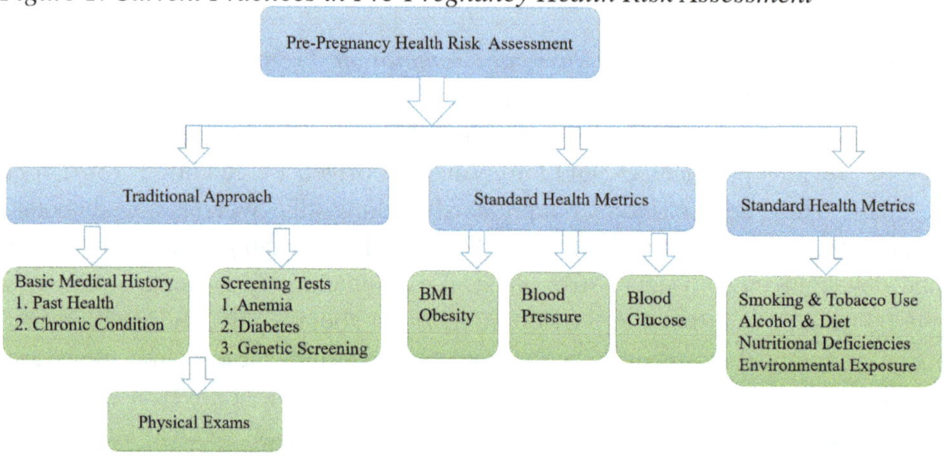

B. Standard Health Metrics

BMI, Blood Pressure, and Blood Glucose Levels: Body Mass Index (BMI), blood pressure, and blood glucose levels are fundamental health metrics that tell a woman's health status concerning pregnancy risks. A high BMI is also a risk factor for gestational diabetes, pre-eclampsia and complications during delivery. One of the essential others is blood pressure, as overly elevated readings can indicate possible hypertension or pre-eclampsia, which can be harmful to mother and child (Bajaj D et al., 2023). Women at risk for gestational diabetes, particularly those with a family history of diabetes, are identified using blood glucose testing. Conception must wait until blood glucose is highly well controlled; uncontrolled diabetes is associated with congenital anomalies and also with other pregnancy complications. These metrics serve as the most standard measurements in traditional screen assessments that healthcare providers use to determine whether interventions prior to conception are necessary (Lipschuetz et al., 2024).

Family History and Genetic Conditions: The family medical history and genetic predisposition are considered for pre-pregnancy assessment. Evaluating a woman's hereditary risk and family history can guide healthcare providers in evaluating her family history to determine if she needs genetic counselling or additional testing (Georgakopoulou V E & Diamanti A, 2024). Hemophilia, cystic fibrosis and some other heart diseases can be identified by family history so couples can make informed reproductive choices. New technological advancements in genetic testing make it possible to test for more things than they used to, now determining whether the person is a disease carrier. The genetic component comes out, and the healthcare provider can give more personal advisory and preventive measures to people with a higher genetic risk (Umans E et al., 2024).

C. Lifestyle Factors

Smoking, Alcohol Consumption, and Diet: Lifestyle choices are associated with pre-pregnancy health as well as subsequent pregnancy outcomes. For instance, smoking can cause healthier risks of miscarriage, decreased birth weight and early birth and employing excessive alcohol enables fetal alcohol spectrum disorders. Getting ready for pregnancy is also essential from the nutrition side since nutritional deficiencies of critical nutrients such as folic acid and iron can cause problems. This includes traditional assessments such as self-reported questionnaires or interviews about lifestyle changes that may be made before pregnancy. Smoking cessation, alcohol avoidance, and dietary change are standard advice to mothers and their babies to improve health (Togunwa T O et al., 2023).

Environmental Exposure: Standard pre-pregnancy screening tests often fail to consult environmental aspects despite these influencing reproductive health and gestational outcomes. Exposure to pesticides, for example, has been associated with an increased risk of miscarriage and congenital anomalies (Patel D J et al., 2024). High birth weights are also associated with high levels of air pollution. Unfortunately, traditional assessments cannot generally capture these environmental exposures due to the complexity and variability of the potential exposures to these risks. Nevertheless, it is crucial to understand such factors in order to give a complete pre-pregnancy risk assessment. For example, pre-pregnancy environmental exposure assessments could help with risks and help promote healthier pregnancies.

2.2 Limitations in Current Practices in Pre-Pregnancy Health Risk Assessment

While conventional procedures are primary to pre-pregnancy health evaluation, they present several limitations, which hinder their effectiveness in exhaustively assuring each individual's health concern. These constraints make apparent the necessity of a more sophisticated, individualized, and inclusive approach to pre-pregnancy care.

Lack of Personalization: Conventional pre-pregnancy health evaluations too often rely on a 'one size fits all' approach regarding an individual's unique health profile. Despite significant variances in genetic background, lifestyle, and individual health history among women, traditional examinations often ignore these variances with standardized approaches. This broad approach may result in the ignoring of risk factors that are specific to each issue for each individual.

Overreliance on Basic Metrics: Basic health metrics such as BMI, blood pressure, and blood glucose levels are the mainstay of conventional prenatal assessments. While these metrics are good proxies of general health status, they often miss the more subtle risk factors. For example, these simple measures might not adequately characterize complex phenotypes affected by generated metabolism and certain lifestyle behaviours. This means that an excessive use of these metrics may hide less apparent health risks that could influence pregnancy outcomes.

Underutilization of Advanced Technologies: Many such advanced technologies like genetic profiling, machine learning algorithms, or real-time health monitoring devices have yet to be used in traditional tests of pre-pregnancy assessment. Machine learning can, for example, mine massive datasets looking for complex patterns and predict an individual's health risks. Genetic profiling would reveal hereditary predispositions and conditions to allow for personalized risk assessments. Conventional practice needs these advanced tools, and with them, the depth and accuracy of assessments are maintained, preventing the use of data-driven insights to inform decision-making better.

Inadequate Focus on Psychosocial Factors: Many such advanced technologies like genetic profiling, machine learning algorithms, or real-time health monitoring devices are yet to be used in the traditional tests of pre-pregnancy assessment. Machine learning can, for example, mine massive datasets looking for complex patterns and predict an individual's health risks. Genetic profiling would reveal hereditary predispositions and conditions to allow for personalized risk assessments. Conventional practice needs these advanced tools, and with them, the depth and accuracy of assessments are maintained, preventing the use of data-driven insights to better inform decision-making.

3. EMERGING TRENDS IN PRE-PREGNANCY HEALTH RISK ASSESSMENT

Now, as healthcare continues to move towards being data-driven and personalized, the emerging trend for pre-pregnancy health risk assessment offers promise for more precise, comprehensive, and individualized care. Achievements in this category include artificial intelligence, genetic knowledge, wearable technologies, and a holistic approach to health that provides better insight into the drivers of pregnancy outcomes.

3.1 Integration of AI and Machine Learning in Pre-Pregnancy Health Risk Assessment

Utilizing Artificial Intelligence (AI) and Machine Learning (ML)-based pre-pregnancy risk assessment represents the game changer that brings the power of advanced computational techniques to reproductive and maternal healthcare. AI and ML models, by analysing vast and complex datasets, give predictive insights to inform early interventions and personalized strategies for care that improve outcomes for mothers and infants. The two technologies in question, in particular, proved very effective at pinpointing risk factors for infertility, maternal health complications and early pregnancy loss, thereby improving accuracy and efficiency in reproductive healthcare. Specific applications and benefits of AI and ML in a pre-pregnancy health risk assessment are presented in the following sections, along with a discussion of the ethical challenges and considerations associated with their implementation.

AI in Fertility Assessment: The utility of AI-powered tools in the field of fertility assessment is also well established, where data pertaining to demographics and clinical are processed by the tools to produce an individualized fertility profile. These tools help by identifying infertility risk factors and predicting fertility potential, thus reducing the diagnostic uncertainty and offering personalized recommendations as to how to apply lifestyle adjustments or use medical intervention for suggested early intervention in reproductive healthcare. Suppose, for example, that AI models could make assessments based on hormonal levels, reproductive history, and lifestyle characteristics and use that information to suggest actions that could help improve fertility. Further, its adaptability allows cycle after cycle of refining the model based on user feedback and research updates (Puri et al., 2024), guaranteeing the relevance and effectiveness of its recommendations in a timely changing medical environment.

Machine Learning in Maternal Health Risk Prediction: Machine learning algorithms predict maternal health risks such as age, blood pressure, glucose levels, and heart rate. For example, these models have been highly accurate when using the Random Forest algorithm with a precision of up to 94.26 percent in predicting risks to maternal health (Thakkar et al., 2024) (Shifa H A. et al., 2024). These ML models come up with buckets (high, medium, and low) to help healthcare professionals allocate resources effectively and provide patients with personalized care depending on their pregnancy risk. Initiating this stratification in optimizing healthcare delivery can focus on the increasing risk of patients, thereby preventing potential complications of pregnancy (Ukrit et al., 2024).

Predictive Modelling for Early Pregnancy Loss: Advanced ML models such as deep learning and multilayer perceptions with high accuracy predict early pregnancy loss (EPL). With these models' variables such as maternal serum vitamin D levels, previous pregnancy outcome, and other clinical markers are evaluated to identify the most crucial determinant of EPL. These predictive models detect women or pregnancies in jeopardy earlier so that interventions during pregnancy can be earlier, hopefully resulting in better pregnancy and gestation health.

AI in Clinical Decision Support: In clinical decision support, AI-driven models are used to predict complications such as preterm birth, gestational diabetes and pre-eclampsia. These models process maternal health data to generate real-time, patient-specific assessments and recommendations that improve prenatal care and reduce the likelihood of adverse outcomes. For example, if an AI model alerts a healthcare provider to early warning signs of pre-eclampsia, he or she can intervene pre-emptively to lessen the risk for both mother and child. Also, AI is used in remote monitoring and telemedicine platforms that increase access to vital healthcare services in remote areas. These platforms allow patients to manage their health away from traditional clinical settings in a continuous, personalized way that better promotes health outcomes (Panda & Sharma, 2024).

Challenges and Considerations

However, the promise of using AI and ML in pre-pregnancy health risk assessment needs to be improved by several challenges that must be addressed to realize their full potential. Key considerations include:

- **Regulatory and Policy Issues**: To integrate AI into healthcare, we need a solid regulatory framework to ensure AI models are safe, reliable, and fair. Clear guidelines must be established for how AI can be used in health assessment to prevent patients from being exposed to risk and assure consistency of practice throughout healthcare.
- **Data Privacy and Security**: Health data is compassionate and requires robust safeguards for the patient's right to privacy. To maintain trust in AI-driven healthcare solutions, it is critical that they comply with data protection regulations, such as GDPR.
- **Ethical and Equity Concerns**: Algorithmic bias in AI systems can result in disparities in healthcare access and outcomes that must be minimized in designing AI systems. Ethical concerns include ensuring equitable access to AI technologies, transparency in AI recommendations, and minimizing unintended biases to promote fair healthcare (Panda P K & Sharma R, 2024).
- **Integration into Clinical Workflows**: However, integrating AI and ML tools into existing clinical workflows can be challenging and necessitates changes to protocols and training for healthcare providers. Our goal is for these technologies to augment, not undermine, clinical decision-making, so seamless integration is required.

3.2 Soft Computing Techniques in Pre-Pregnancy Health Risk Assessment

Figure 2.1 depicts the significant categories of the Soft Computing Techniques used for handling complex, uncertain and imprecise data in computational tasks. The details for these techniques include "Fuzzy Computing (e.g., fuzzy logic) on ambiguity, Neural Networks (e.g., artificial and backpropagation networks) for pattern recognition, and Evolutionary Computing (e.g., genetic algorithms) for optimization and Machine Learning (e.g., supervised and unsupervised learning)" for prediction. Other techniques include chaos theory, belief theory, swarm intelligence (e.g., algorithms inspired by ant colony or particle swarm optimization), and collective behaviour seen in nature. These approaches, in combination, offer flexible, adaptable solutions in data processing and decision-making domains that necessitate intelligent data processing and decision-making Pitkin (2007).

With the capability to handle complex data and manage uncertainty, soft computing techniques, including fuzzy logic, neural networks, and hybrid models, are becoming more valuable in healthcare. These techniques allow us to develop more precise, subtle, and personal evaluations of a woman's health status in pre-pregnancy health risk assessment by processing various complex, uncertain, ambiguous health data. In this section, we study the use of fuzzy logic, neural networks, and hybrid models in pre-assessment.

Fuzzy Logic: Healthcare applications are ideal situations for fuzzy logic due to uncertainty in data. Unlike traditional binary logic systems, fuzzy logic values data along a continuum of values, which are more consistent with real-world health scenarios. In pre-pregnancy health assessments, fuzzy logic can handle subjective and imprecise information as variables, such as lifestyle factors (e.g., physical activity level, dietary habits) and subjective health indicators (e.g. stress level, mental well-being). For instance, rather than thinking of BMI as something that is either normal or overweight, fuzzy logic makes it possible to group BMI into fractions, so that we can ascertain a reasonable range of the potential influence of weight on pregnancy risks. This kind of soft data can be processed and integrated by fuzzy logic to achieve a more flexible and realistic analysis, allowing better pre-pregnancy care decisions (Crider K. S et al. 2022).

Neural Networks: Neural networks, inspired by the structure and functioning of the human brain, are highly effective for pattern recognition and can learn complex relationships within data. In pre-pregnancy risk assessment, neural networks analyze vast amounts of clinical and demographic data to identify intricate patterns that may indicate potential health risks. In particular, these models are very useful for identifying nonlinear relationships with variables (i.e. which combinations (e.g. age + blood pressure + glucose levels. etc.) may increase the chance of complications such as gestational diabetes or preterm birth). Additionally, neural networks are adaptable; they continually improve at predicting accuracy as more data is provided. In pre-pregnancy health assessments, where health data may be diverse and complex, neural networks' ability to work with large, multi-dimensional datasets makes them highly valuable. Neural networks offer insights to identify subtle patterns and connections to offer early intervention and facilitate possibilities of personalized care planning (Diamanti et al., 2019).

Figure 2. Different Soft Computing Techniques

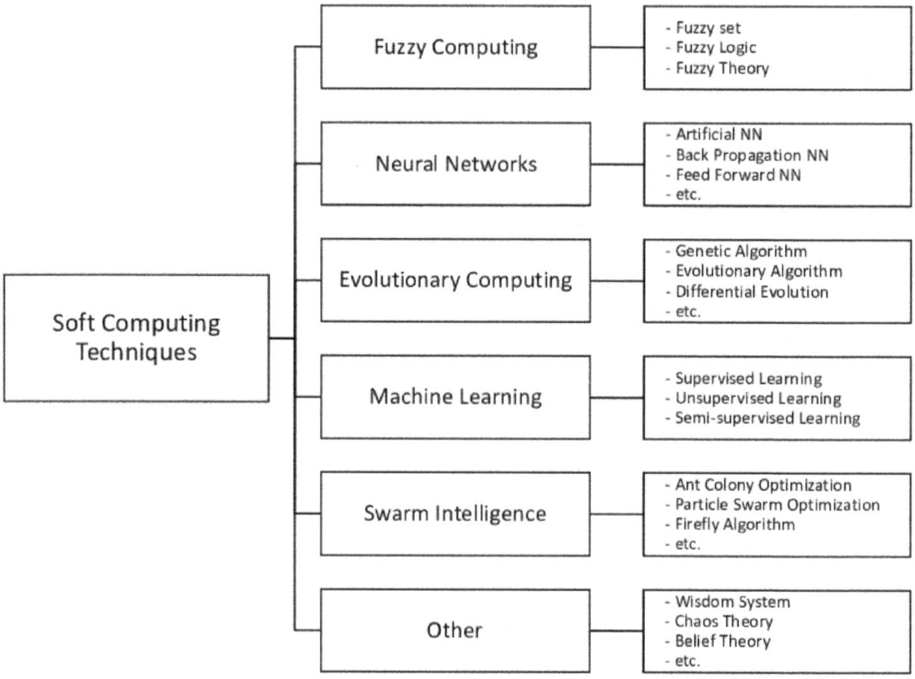

Hybrid Models

Combining Techniques for Enhanced Accuracy: Integrating multiple soft computing techniques is an enhanced method for pre-pregnancy health risk assessment, and such hybrid models combine fuzzy logic with neural networks, for example, expanding the strengths of each technique. Such a hybrid model applies fuzzy logic to process and classify ambiguous or subjective data and neural networks to handle the intricate relationships between health parameters. Take, for example, a hybrid model that first classifies different lifestyle risk factors using fuzzy logic (classification of alcohol intake as 'low,' 'moderate,' or 'high' using fuzzy thresholds), then uses a neural network to analyze how these lifestyle factors relate to clinical data (blood pressure or cholesterol levels) to assess overall pregnancy risk.

Increased Predictive Power and Flexibility: Hybrid modelling approaches improve forecast accuracy and flexibility in handling complicated health data. The hybrid fuzzy neural model would more precisely predict conditions such as gestational diabetes or hypertension, which can effectively represent the complexities involved with individual risk variables and their interaction with the surrounding influences. Additionally, hybrid models will likely improve their predictions continually by continually incorporating increasingly fresh data to increase the accuracy of those predictions over time. Particularly helpful in pre-pregnancy health evaluations, where an individual's health profile could change over time and ongoing research could bring about new risk factors, flexibility is advantageous. By allowing hybrid models to transform disparate data points into heterogeneous data points and deliver highly personalized insights, hybrid models enable proactive and customized pre-pregnancy treatment.

Application of Hybrid Models in Clinical Decision Support: Hybrid models are widely used in clinical decision support to help healthcare professionals form educated and patient-specific recommendations. These models may yield real-time physician evaluations in choosing the most appropriate treatment strategy for each patient by amalgamating fuzzy logic with neural networks. For example, suppose the chosen hybrid model detects a high-risk profile (synthesis of lifestyle variables and clinical data). Specific measures such as dietary adjustments or additional monitoring to prevent potential problems before conception may be suggested in that case. Hybrid models enable healthcare practitioners to provide proactive, tailored pre-pregnancy treatment, delivering improved precision and dependability risk assessments tailored to each patient's unique health profile.

3.3 Wearable and Remote Monitoring Devices in Pre-Pregnancy Health Risk Assessment

The emergence of wearable and remote monitoring technologies fundamentally transforms pre-pregnancy health evaluations by allowing continuous real-time surveillance of vital signs and lifestyle variables, among other health parameters. The data produced by gadgets such as smartwatches, fitness trackers, and specialized health monitors is aggregated and used to evaluate risk effectively and provide tailored health recommendations. Wearables significantly contribute to proactive health management by offering unparalleled access to health information for healthcare practitioners and patients, empowering women to assume a more active role in assuring preparedness for a successful pregnancy.

In Figure 2.3, a Pregnant Woman, a person with wearable sensors on key maternal locations of the body: chest, limb, and abdomen, is shown to monitor vital maternal and fetal health parameters continuously. The chest sensor captures maternal heart rate, respiration rate, and central temperature, valuable maternal cardiovascular and respiratory health indicators. The Limb Sensor usually measures SpO_2 (oxygen saturation) and peripheral temperature, indicating circulatory and oxygenation levels. The abdominal sensor can measure fetal heart rate and uterine contraction, which provides essential information about fetal well-being and labour signs. Together, these sensors enable real-time, non-invasive tracking of the fundamental health indicators. They can present a window into the health of both mother and baby as unique identifiers.

Figure 3. Overview of the maternal-fetal monitoring system

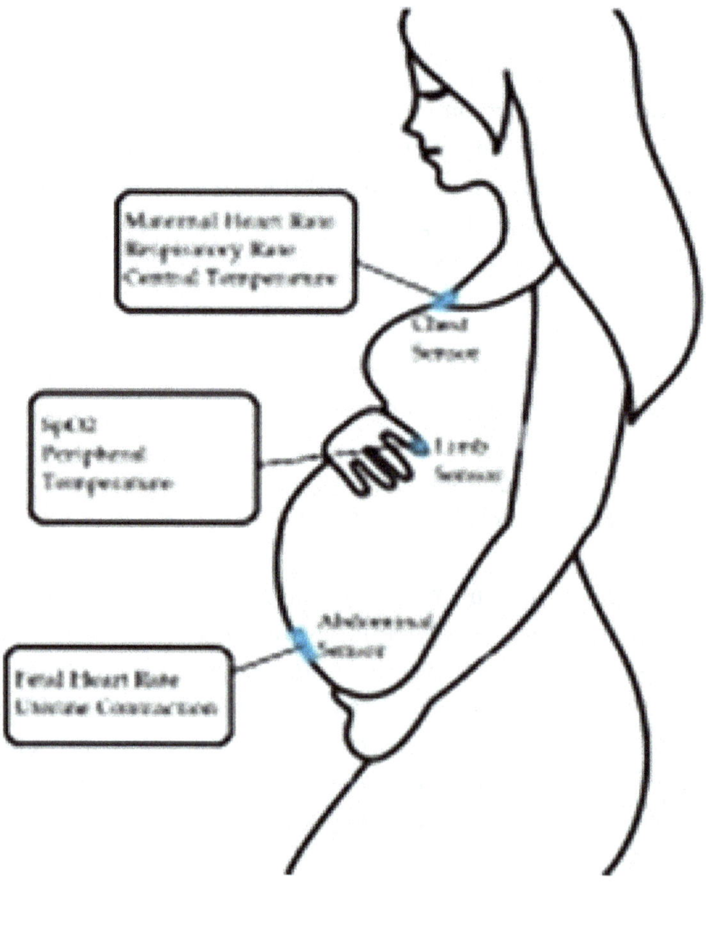

A. Continuous Health Monitoring

Real-Time Data Collection and Analysis: Continuous monitoring of important health parameters, including heart rate, blood pressure, blood oxygen levels, and physical activity, can be achieved using wearable devices. This real-time data is collected, giving a more comprehensive view of women's health compared to assessments in a clinical setting each cycle. Wearables can help you identify trends in your health, early warning signs like, it might be your heart rate changing daily to high to point the stress, your sleep pattern still the same or your physical activity level lower than before, showing that something might be wrong. This continuous flow of data in pre-pregnancy assessment helps healthcare providers know a patient's baseline health and detect possible risk factors for pregnancy complications at the earliest possible opportunity. For example, continuous monitoring of physical activity levels and sleep patterns may uncover lifestyle habits that impact pre-pregnancy health, thus enabling early interventions and recommendations for lifestyle improvements.

Improved Accuracy in Risk Assessment: Real-time data significantly improves the accuracy of pre-pregnancy risk assessments. Because Wearables give us detailed, continuous data points, we are less reliant on self-reported, which needs to be completed or updated. The detailed data provides healthcare providers a better means of making more precise assessments, including whether blood pressure or heart rate fluctuations lie on the healthier side of the spectrum. Wearable devices provide real-time insights that enable dynamic risk assessment in which recommendations can be changed based on the patient's current health status, not their past data. It helps healthcare providers make data-informed decisions and provides a finer understanding of the patient's health profile to give better targeted and effective pre-pregnancy care.

B. Patient Empowerment

Enhanced Awareness of Health Status: Patients are empowered by wearable devices because they can continuously have access to their health metrics. In conjunction with real-time feedback on vital signs and lifestyle factors, women can become more aware of their health status and make informed decisions regarding their daily habits. For example, watching a person's daily activity levels or following sleep quality might inspire someone to become less sedentary or improve her sleep regimen. For example, wearables enable users to create personal goals, have personalized reminders about medication or hydration, and track their progress over time, giving users a sense of ownership over their health. Active engagement with one's health data helps patients proactively manage their health and achieve better outcomes during pregnancy.

Proactive Health Management: The data provided by wearable devices empowers women to do things proactively before they become severe and helps them adjust to being healthier women. Suppose a wearable device detects an ongoing pattern of high-stress levels; then, a patient can respond to stress through mindfulness, relaxation exercises, or lifestyle changes. In pre-pregnancy care, this proactive approach is precious because it is essential to preserve optimal health before conception and reduce risks during pregnancy. Women can help make more timely changes to establish a healthier pregnancy by continuously monitoring their health. Wearable devices allow two-way communication with healthcare providers via data sharing to enable informed conversations and collaborative decisions.

3.4 Comparative Analysis of Traditional and Emerging Approaches in Pre-Pregnancy Health Risk Assessment

An analysis of how pre-pregnancy health risk assessment is being developed provides insight into the differences in accuracy, personalization, data utilization, and practicality between traditional and emerging approaches. This analysis highlights the factors that impact the positive and negative aspects of integrating cutting-edge technologies, such as Artificial Intelligence, Machine Learning, and soft computing, into conventional process processes.

Table 1. Comparison of Traditional and Emerging Approaches in Pre-Pregnancy Health Risk Assessment

Aspect	Traditional Approaches	Emerging Approaches (AI et al., Advanced Technologies)
Accuracy and Reliability	It relies on basic metrics and standardized assessments, leading to generalized and sometimes limited accuracy.	Utilizes advanced algorithms (e.g., machine learning, fuzzy logic) for high accuracy and adaptability in identifying subtle and complex risk factors.
Personalization	Applies a "one-size-fits-all" approach, often resulting in generalized recommendations for all patients.	Offers highly personalized assessments by analyzing individual health characteristics, such as genetic information and lifestyle factors.
Data Utilization	It is limited to essential health data sources, such as medical history, BMI, and blood pressure measurements.	Integrates diverse data sources, including real-time data from wearables, genetic profiling, and environmental data, for a comprehensive view.

continued on following page

Table 1. Continued

Aspect	Traditional Approaches	Emerging Approaches (AI et al., Advanced Technologies)
Psychosocial Factors	Often limited or lacks focus on psychosocial elements like mental health, stress, and social support.	It can incorporate psychosocial metrics, such as mental health assessments and stress monitoring, to provide a holistic view of health.
Predictive Capability	Limited predictive ability, often only identifying immediate, obvious health risks.	High predictive power through machine learning models, which analyze large datasets to predict potential pregnancy complications proactively.
Scalability and Accessibility	Widely accessible, low-cost, and suitable for broad populations, including low-resource settings.	Currently, it is more expensive and infrastructure-intensive; however, costs are expected to decrease with technological advancements.
Implementation Complexity	Simple to implement, often requiring minimal training for healthcare providers.	It is more complex to implement, and specialized tools (e.g., genetic testing, wearable devices) and trained professionals are needed for interpretation.
Adaptability and Learning	Static, relying on fixed guidelines that may not evolve with new medical knowledge.	Adaptive through continuous learning and updates, as machine learning models improve with access to new data and evolving healthcare standards.
Cost Considerations	Generally low-cost, with fewer resources and technology requirements.	There is a higher initial cost due to advanced technology, though long-term costs may be reduced as AI and soft computing become more accessible.

3.5 Challenges and Future Directions in Pre-Pregnancy Health Risk Assessment

As advanced technologies like AI and soft computing become integral to pre-pregnancy health risk assessment, several challenges and future research directions must be addressed to ensure ethical, accessible, and practical care.

1. **Data Privacy and Security**: Privacy and security are paramount as personal health data becomes increasingly woven into AI-driven assessments. Sensitive information about pre-pregnancy assessments, which includes genetic data, medical history, and lifestyle details, must be protected from unauthorized access and misuse, as advanced pre-pregnancy assessments rely on it. This necessitates robust encryption, secure storage systems, and tight controls on access. We also need clear policies around data ownership, consent, and transparency to build patient trust. Future solutions should put data security first, respecting established data protection standards such as GDPR while assuring that personal information is kept safe in the healthcare sector.

2. **Ethical and Regulatory Challenges**: When applied in practice, AI in healthcare raises ethical challenges, most notably around fairness, transparency and accountability. However, if the data used to train models isn't diverse, AI algorithms may inadvertently introduce bias, potentially decreasing the accuracy of the assessment for specific populations. In addition, regulatory frameworks are needed to regulate the ethical use of AI in healthcare, adapting the use of these systems in a transparent and accountable manner. There should be regulations that involve the responsibilities of healthcare providers and AI developers for diagnosis and treatment prescriptions. Therefore, regulatory bodies must set guidelines to ensure that AI-driven assessments meet ethical standards and provide and are being used as decision support, not as definitive diagnostic authorities.
3. **Cost and Accessibility**: Advanced technology in pre-pregnancy care can be costly and might reduce access for patients in low-resource settings. A significant amount of investment is needed not only to implement AI systems, genetic testing, and wearable devices but also an initial investment and additional maintenance, updating and training of healthcare providers. We also need to consider how the high cost may lead to disparities in access since only some healthcare facilities or regions can afford these technologies. This should focus on the cost efficiency and scalability of these technologies that will be developed in the future. It could mean developing cheap AI models and making advanced pre-pregnancy care accessible to a more extensive population through services or partnerships with governments or NGOs.
4. **Interdisciplinary Collaboration**: Pre-pregnancy health risk assessment needs collaboration from healthcare providers, data scientists, policymakers, and technology developers. Healthcare providers provide expertise in clinical subject matter, and data scientists bring analytical skills to create accurate AI models. Policymakers and technology developers work on creating supportive regulatory environments while designing a user-friendly solution which quickly and seamlessly fits into healthcare systems. Interdisciplinary collaboration is required to develop comprehensive, practical and ethical solutions to the complexities of pre-pregnancy care. This can also result in the setting up of standard protocols, allowing for a sharing culture and ensuring that all services work on the same moot point for the processes in the other sectors that go into pre-pregnancy-pre-pregnancy healthcare.
5. **Future Research Directions**: There are several areas for future research to improve pre-pregnancy health risk assessments. Enhancing more complicated AI systems to decode diverse and complicated health data is the key to enhancing prediction accuracy. The inclusion of other parameters which are psychosocial, such as stress levels, mental status and measures of social support, would provide

a more global perspective on a woman's health. Further, refining wearable technology for constant, könnte-wear monitoring will give individuals a better view into and ability to manage their risk profile. One potential direction for future work is the development of new methods for building so-called 'explainable' AI (XAI), which makes the decision-making process more transparent and allows clinicians and patients to understand better why an AI-based recommendation was given. Together, these research directions can help improve the field's individualized, accurate, and ethical pre-conception health evaluation.

4. CONCLUSION

This review outlines the advances and limitations of pre-pregnancy health risk assessment practices and argues for more personalized, accurate and comprehensive approaches. While foundational, traditional methods are not precise or deep enough to discover the entire spectrum of risk factors affecting maternal and fetal health. The existing technologies like artificial intelligence, soft computing and genomic profiling offer the colossal potential to realize predictive modelling, data-driven personalization and data integration from disparate sources such as genetic and real-time health. Health outcomes will improve if these innovations can lead to more precise assessments and tailored recommendations. This potential is dependent on more research, an unprecedented level of interdisciplinary collaboration and investment in the highest quality, most accessible, ethical and practical technologies. Fill these gaps, and future innovations can provide robust, personalized pre-pregnancy health solutions that enable women and their physicians to have safer, healthier pregnancies.

REFERENCES

Bajaj, D., Kumari, R., & Bansal, P. (2023). Risk level prediction for maternal health using machine learning algorithms. In *2023 International Conference on Communication, Security and Artificial Intelligence (ICCSAI)* (pp. 405-409). IEEE.

Crider, K. S., Qi, Y. P., & Yeung, L. F.. (2022). Folic acid and the prevention of birth defects: 30 years of opportunity and controversies. *Annual Review of Nutrition, 42*, 423–452. PMID: 35995050

Diamanti, A., Papadakis, S., & Schoretsaniti, S.. (2019). Smoking cessation in pregnancy: An update for maternity care practitioners. *Tobacco Induced Diseases, 17*, 57. PMID: 31582946

Georgakopoulou, V. E., & Diamanti, A. (2024). Artificial intelligence for smoking cessation in pregnancy. *Cureus, 16*(7). PMID: 39100043

Lipschuetz, M., Guedalia, J., Cohen, S. M., Unger, R., Yagel, S., & Sompolinsky, Y. (2024). Machine learning in electronic health records: Identifying high-risk obstetric patients pre and during labor. In *Innovation in Applied Nursing Informatics* (pp. 3–7). IOS Press.

Lipschuetz, M., Guedalia, J., Cohen, S. M., Unger, R., Yagel, S., & Sompolinsky, Y. (2024). Machine learning in electronic health records: Identifying high-risk obstetric patients pre and during labor. In *Innovation in Applied Nursing Informatics* (pp. 3–7). IOS Press.

Panda, P. K., & Sharma, R. (2024). Transforming maternal healthcare: Harnessing the power of artificial intelligence for improved outcomes and access. *World Journal of Advanced Research and Reviews, 23*(1), 662–666.

Parveen, G., Joshi, P., Uniyal, Y., & Rawat, S. (2024). Contribution of artificial intelligence to improving women's health in pregnancy. In *Artificial Intelligence and Machine Learning for Women's Health Issues* (pp. 121–135). Academic Press.

Patel, D. J., Chaudhari, K., Acharya, N., Shrivastava, D., & Muneeba, S. (2024). Artificial intelligence in obstetrics and gynecology: Transforming care and outcomes. *Cureus, 16*(7), e64725. PMID: 39156405

Pitkin, R. M. (2007). Folate and neural tube defects. *The American Journal of Clinical Nutrition, 85*, 285S–288S. PMID: 17209211

Puri, A., Mathur, R., & Nayar, K. D. (2024). AI-powered fertility assessment tool. *International Journal of Science and Research Archive, 12*(1), 742–744.

Raihen, M. N., & Akter, S. (2024). Comparative assessment of several effective machine learning classification methods for maternal health risk. *Computational Journal of Mathematical and Statistical Sciences*, *3*(1), 161–176.

Shifa, H. A., Mojumdar, M. U., Rahman, M. M., Chakraborty, N. R., & Gupta, V. (2024). Machine learning models for maternal health risk prediction based on clinical data. In *2024 11th International Conference on Computing for Sustainable Global Development (INDIACom)* (pp. 1312-1318). IEEE.

Sufian, M. A., Hamzi, W., Hamzi, B., Sagar, A. S., Rahman, M., Varadarajan, J., Hanumanthu, M., & Azad, M. A. K. (2024). Innovative machine learning strategies for early detection and prevention of pregnancy loss: The vitamin D connection and gestational health. *Diagnostics (Basel)*, *14*(9), 920. PMID: 38732334

Sufian, M. A., Hamzi, W., Hamzi, B., Sagar, A. S., Rahman, M., Varadarajan, J., Hanumanthu, M., & Azad, M. A. K. (2024). Innovative machine learning strategies for early detection and prevention of pregnancy loss: The vitamin D connection and gestational health. *Diagnostics (Basel)*, *14*(9), 920. PMID: 38732334

Swathikrishna, M. R., Sriram, S., & Subha, B. (2023). Pre-eclampsia risk prediction using machine learning algorithms. In *International Conference on Information and Communication Technology for Competitive Strategies* (pp. 71-80). Singapore: Springer Nature Singapore.

Thakkar, D., Gandhi, V. C., & Trivedi, D. (2024). Forecasting maternal women's health risks using random forest classifier. In *2024 International Conference on Inventive Computation Technologies (ICICT)* (pp. 961-965). IEEE.

Tiwari, R. G., Agarwal, A. K., & Jain, V. (2023). Leveraging machine learning for comprehensive analysis of maternal health: Predicting health risks and improving antenatal care. In *International Conference on Mobile Radio Communications & 5G Networks* (pp. 287-297). Singapore: Springer Nature Singapore.

Togunwa, T. O., Babatunde, A. O., & Abdullah, K. (2023). Deep hybrid model for maternal health risk classification in pregnancy: Synergy of ANN and random forest. *Frontiers in Artificial Intelligence*, *6*, 1213436. PMID: 37476504

Ukrit, M. F., Jeyavathana, R. B., Rani, A. L., & Chandana, V. (2024). Maternal health risk prediction with machine learning methods. In *2024 Second International Conference on Emerging Trends in Information Technology and Engineering (ICE-TITE)* (pp. 1-9). IEEE.

Umans, E., Dewilde, K., Williams, H., Deprest, J., & Van den Bosch, T. (2024). Artificial intelligence in imaging in the first trimester of pregnancy: A systematic review. *Fetal Diagnosis and Therapy*, *51*(4), 343–356. PMID: 38493764

Yaseen, I., & Rather, R. A. (2024). A theoretical exploration of artificial intelligence's impact on feto-maternal health from conception to delivery. *International Journal of Women's Health*, •••, 903–915. PMID: 38800118

Chapter 4
Revolutionizing Brain Tumor Detection by Exploring the Environmental Impact and Deep Learning in MRI Segmentation

Snehal Rahul Rathi
https://orcid.org/0009-0004-7638-6429
Vishwakarma Institute of Information Technology, Pune, India

Pratik Kanhaiya Rathod
Vishwakarma Institute of Information Technology, Pune, India

Adarsh R. Dawkhare
Vishwakarma Institute of Information Technology, Pune, India

Sanket Sunil Anbhule
https://orcid.org/0009-0004-7807-7435
Vishwakarma Institute of Information Technology, Pune, India

Shilpa Prashant Kalantri
https://orcid.org/0000-0002-7011-2513
Shah and Anchor Kutchhi Engineering College, India

DOI: 10.4018/979-8-3373-0179-2.ch004

t © 2026, IGI Global Scientific Publishing. Copying or distributing in print or electronic forms without written permission of IGI Global Scientific Publishing is prohibited. Use of this chapter to enerative artificial intelligence (AI) technologies is expressly prohibited. The publisher reserves all rights to license its use for generative AI training and machine learning model development.

ABSTRACT

Maligancy of the brain is a disorder that affects the health of populations worldwide and for diagnosis, calls for complex skills and high-resolution techniques. This work proposes the use of a new strategy for the detection and segmentation of brain tumors with the help of MRI images. Concerning MRI, although the tumors are high in water content and possess hydrogen atoms, they give variations in signal intensity when compared to normal tissues. Thus, the utilization of CNNs for classifying and detecting brain tumors is quite efficient, provided the combined application of the CLAHE algorithm to boost the image contrast, where the outcomes of the classification attained a high accuracy. This chapter reflects on the Sustainable Development Goals in general by contributing to the development of more effective diagnostic tools and, consequently, enhancing the health of individuals. It is in line with the need to have sustainable healthcare systems for the constant and fair diagnosis and treatment of brain tumors regardless of the climate situation.

INTRODUCTION

The brain has an amazing number of cells and is one of the finest-built organs of the human body. Brain tumor is one of the main reasons for the growth of human demise. The brain tumor is an abnormal growth of the cells which are known as cancerous tumor or also known as a malignant tumor (Kumar et al., 2021). Tumors can occur where they start in one area and continue to grow, or they begin and develop at the same location in other tissues. This form of tumor is said to be the primary tumor; it is said that it cannot differentiate from other areas like spreading. The brain, with its astonishing number of neurons, stands as one of the most intricately designed organs in the human body. Brain tumors represent a significant cause of mortality, marked by abnormal cell growth, known as malignant or cancerous tumors. Tumors can either initiate in a singular location and proliferate or emerge and expand within the same tissue region. These are classified as primary tumors, distinguished by their non-metastatic nature.

Among the most frequently diagnosed brain tumors are gliomas, meningiomas, pituitary adenomas, medulloblastomas, and schwannomas. Although the precise etiology of brain tumors remains elusive, several factors are believed to contribute, including high radiation exposure, various genetic conditions, and a compromised immune system, particularly in younger individuals. The clinical manifestations of brain tumors vary with their size and location but commonly include headaches, seizures, visual or auditory impairments, limb weakness or numbness, and difficulties with speech or movement. Diagnostic methods typically involve a combination of imaging techniques, such as biopsies, MRI scans, and other advanced imaging technologies. The MRI, utilizing radio waves and potent magnetic fields, offers a detailed visualization of the brain's internal structures, aiding in the detection of anomalies. Given the significant impact of brain tumors on global health, accurate and timely diagnosis is crucial. This study introduces a pioneering approach to brain tumor identification and MRI segmentation, leveraging the unique characteristics of tumors, notably the higher water concentration and excess hydrogen atoms, which create distinct intensity variations in MRI images.

Gliomas, Meningiomas, Pituitary adenomas, Medullobla-stomas, Schwannomas were the most commonly reported brain tumors from patients. It is unclear what causes a brain tumor, but many issues are believed to influence the tumor. These are the high radiation dosage, a number of genetic disorders, and a person's weak defense against an adolescent or youthful brain tumor diagnosed. The symptoms of brain tumors change depending on the location and size, but common indications are headache, epilepsy, blurred or obscured vision or hearing loss, weakening or numbness in limbs, or difficulty speaking or moving. The combination of imaging tests such as removing a tiny amount of brain tumor tissue for testing with a machine that cuts into the brain and MRIs, a medical imaging procedure that uses radio waves and strong magnetic fields to produce a precise photograph of organs, are usually utilized in the identification. The incidence of brain tumors has steadily increased, posing significant challenges to the medical community. Accurate and timely diagnosis is vital for effective treatment, yet traditional methods often fall short due to the complex nature of brain anatomy and tumor characteristics. This paper aims to address this gap by leveraging deep learning techniques, particularly Convolutional Neural Networks (CNNs), to improve the accuracy of brain tumor detection through MRI segmentation. Our approach integrates state-of-the-art algorithms with advanced image processing techniques, offering a promising solution to this critical healthcare issue.

As an instrumental cause of global mortality and morbidity, brain tumors call for specialized experience and state-of-the-art imaging technologies for proper diagnosis. Notably, the study presents a novel approach to brain tumor identification and magnetic resonance imaging segmentation. It is based on the distinct characteristic of tumors in MRI, where the high-water concentration, and excess of hydrogen atoms contrast the variations in intensity of the MRI image between a normal and tumor area. The signs of brain tumors may also be disturbing, they might resemble the symptoms of a few other diseases or any other. The particular kind, site, and size of the brain tumor, as well as the individual's overall health, all determine the available treatment alternatives. Examples include radiotherapy, medicines, surgery, or a mix of many of these techniques. In 2020, the International Agency for Research on Cancer reported 280,000 new cases of brain and neurological disorders worldwide. Through the combination of CLAHE for contrast enhancement and CNN for feature identification, the resulting methodology demonstrates an impressive 98% accuracy for brain tumor detection through MRI. Therefore, deep learning calls for the promotion of enhanced accurate perceptions that may considerably enhance the quality of investigations for patients present. Brain tumors are one of the most complex and difficult-to-diagnose diseases. The subtlety of the human brain combined with the subtlety of tumors often makes them quite elusive for correct detection. However, the advent of deep learning in MRI segmentation will completely revolutionize this area and bring new hope to patients and doctors alike. This chapter discusses the transforming potential of deep learning technologies in brain tumor detection and how they can enhance accuracy, reduce human errors, and ultimately improve patient outcomes.

The American Brain Tumor Association estimates that in 2022, thousands of new cases of primary brain tumors were diagnosed, including both benign and malignant forms. Because of its intricate anatomy and composition, the brain is known to be cancer-resistant. The current brain tumor diagnosis methods are for the most part semiautomatic and are depending on the individual superfluous to decision-making that they render during the MRI checking and this increases the false-positive, Edison's nose, and increased failure of brain tumor identification among other risks for the equipment, since the danger of the huge level noise presented in MRI images. Various proposals for system enhancement suggest that systems based on machine learning and other mechanization are not beneficial because they handle limited data. This chapter proposes a method that is fully automatic. The machine learning classification technique utilizes the fundamental property of Magnetic Resonance Images called 'Intensity Difference.' This characteristic is employed by the CNN algorithm to categorize MRI images. This automatic system has three phases.

i. Image Pre-Processing: Noise Reduction from MRI images.
ii. Image segmentation – To find a region of the image that has a tumor.
iii. Image Post-processing: Extraction of brain Tumor. The CNN algorithm is one of the best algorithms in image segmentation, and it is used in the suggested paper, and it is also excellent for identifying patterns and features in images. That mustn't be extracted manually.

This chapter is organized in various sections which includes literature survey, methodology, algorithm, applications, limitations and future scope.

LITERATURE REVIEW

Kunar et al. (2021) go over the approaches and conclusions of 20 studies on the identification and classification of brain cancers from MRI images that were published between 2000 and 2020.The use of CNN classification techniques is found to be effective for accurately detecting brain tumors with a low error rate. The review suggests that future work should focus on improving accuracy and reducing errors using different classifier techniques. Overall, the potential of automated methods for enhancing brain tumor identification and therapy is highlighted by this review of the research. Three steps make up the novel approach to brain tumor identification put out by Gobhinath et al. (2021) 1) picture pre-processing, 2) image segmentation, and 3) image morphological function. The proposed method uses wavelet transform and PCA to acquire the image features of a tumor and KSVM (kernel support vector machine) to classify the tumor. When the suggested approach was used to 240 MRI scan pictures of the human brain, encompassing seven general brain illnesses, it produced a 98.17% classification accuracy using the GTB kernel. The results of this study indicate that the proposed PCA+DWT+KSVM method with the GTB kernel provides accurate classification and feature extraction output.

Ali et al. (2020) focus on using deep learning algorithms to accurately segment brain tumors from medical images. The two segmentation networks proposed in the paper are 1) 3D CNN and 2) U-Net. The BRATS-19 challenge dataset is used to train the system that is suggested in this research. These networks' outputs are integrated into a method that produces more precise and superior tumor tissue type predictions. The proposed ensemble achieved good dice scores on the validation set, outperforming state-of-the-art techniques. The paper also analyzed different ensemble techniques to determine which is the most accurate. The results showed that the proposed ensemble scheme is better than simple average. Vaishnavee & Amshakala (2015) proposed HFS-SOM for segmentation and PSVM for the classification of brain MRI images. GLCM-PCA is employed for feature extraction and selection. The system achieves high accuracy and less error rates for normal and abnormal brain classification. The study highlights the importance of accurate medical image processing for disease diagnosis, particularly brain tumor detection.

An enhanced U-net model is put forth by Yang & Song (2018) for the automatic segmentation of MRI images of brain tumors. To solve the unbalanced data distribution problem the method uses a patches-based input and introduces a feature recombination layer to shorten training time and reduce training parameters. The study evaluates the proposed algorithm is using the HGG dataset of the Brats 2015 training set using a five-fold cross-validation method, demonstrating strong competitiveness compared to other convolutional network models. However, the evaluation is limited to the HGG dataset, and traditional data augmentation methods are not used, indicating the need for further research to validate the proposed method's performance on other datasets and address the unbalanced data distribution problem.

The paper "Tumor Detection in the Brain using Faster R-CNN" by Ezhilarasi and Varalakshmi (2018) presented at the Proceedings of the Second International Conference on I-SMAC (IoT in Social, Mobile, Analytics, and Cloud) in 2018, explores an innovative method for detecting brain tumors using the Faster R-CNN deep learning architecture. This research provides valuable insights into the effectiveness of Faster R-CNN in accurately identifying brain tumors, contributing to the broader understanding of its applications in medical imaging and diagnostics. The paper titled "An Algorithmic Detection of Brain Tumor Using Image Filtering and Segmentation of Various Radiographs," authored by Mahesh Swami and Divya Verma, (2020) was presented at the 2020 7th International Conference on Signal Processing and Integrated Networks (SPIN). This research explores the development of an innovative algorithm designed to detect brain tumors through advanced image filtering and segmentation techniques applied to various radiographs. The paper significantly contributes to the field by proposing novel methodologies in image processing, aimed at enhancing the accuracy and efficiency of brain tumor detection.

Kaur & Sharma (2017) describe a self-adaptive K-means clustering algorithm that requires no user input for the number of clusters and can accurately detect brain cancers with a short execution time. The segmented portion is converted into a binary image for the purpose of estimating size and position. The gray version is then utilized to extract textural and color-based elements for growth analysis. Size estimation is applied to the final divided section using perimeter and area metrics. Every MRI slice that the algorithm finds shows the growth of a brain tumor, and the graphical profile of the tumor's perimeter and area is constant. The algorithm could potentially be used to compute tumor growth in the blood oxygen area during fMRI for the state of brain analysis. A brain tumor identification system utilizing an artificial neural network (ANN) and support vector machine (SVM) is proposed by Kabir et al. (2020). On the BRATS dataset, the algorithm, which consists of stages like image enhancement, segmentation, feature extraction, and classification, has a 97.7% accuracy rate. The neural network uses a fully connected backpropagation model with 40 neurons in the hidden layer and a tanh activation function. The proposed algorithm provides better accuracy than existing methods and can be further improved by incorporating convolutional neural networks for larger datasets.

The application of diagnostic imaging for medical analysis and brain tumor identification is covered by Dhanve & Kumar (2017). The authors suggest a novel approach to brain tumor identification that combines object labeling algorithms for tumor area recognition with k-means partitioning. The proposed technique involves preprocessing using a median filter and morphological operation to remove noise and the skull part of the brain. The paper provides a detailed explanation of each stage of the proposed system, including algorithms used and results obtained. Chandra & Bajpai (2018) present a new fractional mask design for detecting benign brain tumors, which addresses the limitations of existing techniques. A numerical head phantom is used to test the suggested approach, and it is compared to well-known boundary-based techniques including Sobel, Prewitt, Canny, and Laplacian of Gaussian (LoG). The results show that the fractional order mask is superior to existing methods and is able to detect small intensity variations in the image. The performance of the suggested strategy is also assessed quantitatively, indicating that it is successful in identifying benign brain tumors. A technique to identify and categorize brain tumors as benign or malignant is put forth by Hebli & Gupta (2017). The proposed methodology involves pre-processing the MR image, segmenting the tumor using morphological operations, extracting tumor features using Discrete Wavelet Transform (DWT), and classifying the tumor using Support Vector Machine (SVM). The image is first pre-processed by resizing and converting to grayscale, followed by morphological operations. To categorize a tumor as benign or malignant, characteristics are extracted from the image using the DWT and fed into SVM classifiers. Al-Galal et al.'s (2021) systematic review fits within a broader context of research exploring the application of deep learning techniques to medical imaging, particularly for the analysis of MRI brain tumor images. Previous studies have employed various deep learning architectures, each contributing unique insights and advancements to the field. Here, we highlight key comparative studies and their relevance to the findings of Al-Galal et al.

Rahman et al.'s (2022) work fits into a growing body of research that explores the intersection of IoT and medical diagnostics. Prior studies have demonstrated the feasibility of IoT in various healthcare applications, including remote patient monitoring and chronic disease management. However, the application of IoT specifically for brain tumor detection remains relatively novel. Compared to previous approaches that primarily focus on image analysis using standalone systems, Rahman et al.'s IoT-based system offers the advantage of connectivity and real-time data processing. This connectivity facilitates continuous monitoring and quick diagnostic responses, which are critical in managing conditions like brain tumors. The work of Ayadi et al. (2021) fits within a broader body of research focused on the application of deep learning to medical image analysis. Previous studies have explored various CNN architectures and training strategies for brain tumor classification, with varying degrees of success. For example, earlier works often employed shallower networks or hybrid approaches combining CNNs with traditional machine learning classifiers. Ayadi et al.'s deep CNN model represents a significant advancement over these earlier methods. By employing a deeper network architecture, they are able to capture more detailed and complex features from MRI images, leading to improved classification performance. Additionally, their comprehensive evaluation on a diverse dataset provides strong evidence of the model's generalizability.

The issue of automatically identifying brain cancers in MRI images using deep learning models is covered by Ayadi et al. (2021). The current state-of-the-art model uses a CNN with small convolution kernels, which has shown significant improvement in accuracy, specificity, and sensitivity while reducing processing time. To address these limitations, the authors propose a DNN model that includes modifications in the segmentation and feature-extraction stages. They used only 10 MRI images to train the model and to check its performance which is too less. Validation of the model with a larger dataset is recommended also there may be a decrease in response time & decline in the performance of the model when trained on a larger dataset. Ahmed & Sabir (2015) In this paper used Hidden Markov Random Fields (HMRF) model. These models have been widely proposed for segmenting homogeneous and noisy regions in MR images. The EM algorithm is commonly employed in this context to estimate the parameters of pertinent probabilistic models. The proposed method achieved good results for segmenting glioma tumors. In the diagnosis of brain tumors, hybrid approaches combining HMRF and thresholding techniques have also demonstrated encouraging outcomes.

By looking at the literature survey, it has been observed that there is a need of the system having enhanced diagnostic capabilities and user-friendly interface. Brief description of it is as follows.

1. Enhanced Diagnostic Capabilities

- The integration of Convolutional Neural Networks (CNNs) into medical imaging has orchestrated a revolutionary upheaval in the domain, bestowing upon its unparalleled levels of precision in the identification and categorization of tumors. Unlike archaic methodologies heavily contingent upon human proficiency, CNNs possess the innate capacity to autonomously assimilate and distill salient attributes from MRI scans, thereby mitigating the susceptibility to human fallibility and amplifying diagnostic acumen. Moreover, the assimilation of Contrast Limited Adaptive Histogram Equalization (CLAHE) serves to augment the fidelity of images, thereby expediting the early detection of tumors when therapeutic intervention is maximally efficacious.

2. Comprehensive Image Processing Pipeline

Our envisioned system endeavors to harness a multifaceted image processing pipeline meticulously crafted to optimize the efficacy of tumor detection. This encompasses:

a. **Image Pre-processing:** Refining the quality of MRI scans through methodologies such as median filtering and CLAHE, which ameliorate visibility and abate noise.
b. **Image Segmentation:** Harnessing global thresholding to delineate the tumor region, thereby facilitating more precise analysis.
c. **Feature Extraction:** Employing CNN windowing techniques to glean pertinent features from segmented images, pivotal for meticulous classification.
d. **Image Classification:** Leveraging sophisticated machine learning algorithms such as SVM and k-NN to stratify MRI images, discerning the presence of tumors.

3. User-Friendly Interface

In a bid to ensure the accessibility of our system to healthcare practitioners, we have endeavored to fashion an intuitive interface employing React.js and Flask. This interface affords users the convenience of effortlessly uploading MRI images and expeditiously receiving predictive outputs concerning tumor detection and classification. Such user-friendliness serves to democratize access to advanced diagnostic capabilities, thereby rendering them accessible even to healthcare establishments with finite resources.

METHODOLOGY

Our investigation endeavors to discern cerebral neoplasms from medical imagery, employing a methodology that encompasses several stages. These stages comprise preprocessing, segmentation, feature extraction, and classification. The principal aim of image preprocessing is to refine the caliber of medical visuals, rendering them tidier and more conducive for further scrutiny. Segmentation assumes a pivotal role in segregating the tumorous locus from the adjacent cerebral tissues. This undertaking is indispensable for precise identification and assessment of the neoplasm. Subsequent processing entails morphological maneuvers that further hone the segmented area, ensuring heightened precision in tumor discernment.

Feature extraction constitutes a cardinal process wherein CNN windowing techniques are deployed to extricate pivotal attributes from the medical visuals. These attributes are pivotal in demarcating between neoplastic and non-neoplastic territories. Lastly, classification stratifies the medical visuals into two cohorts: those devoid of neoplasms and those with neoplasms. This step is pivotal in furnishing actionable insights for healthcare practitioners, facilitating prompt and efficacious therapeutic determination. Figure 1 displays the flow of steps used during model training.

Figure 1. Process flow of the system

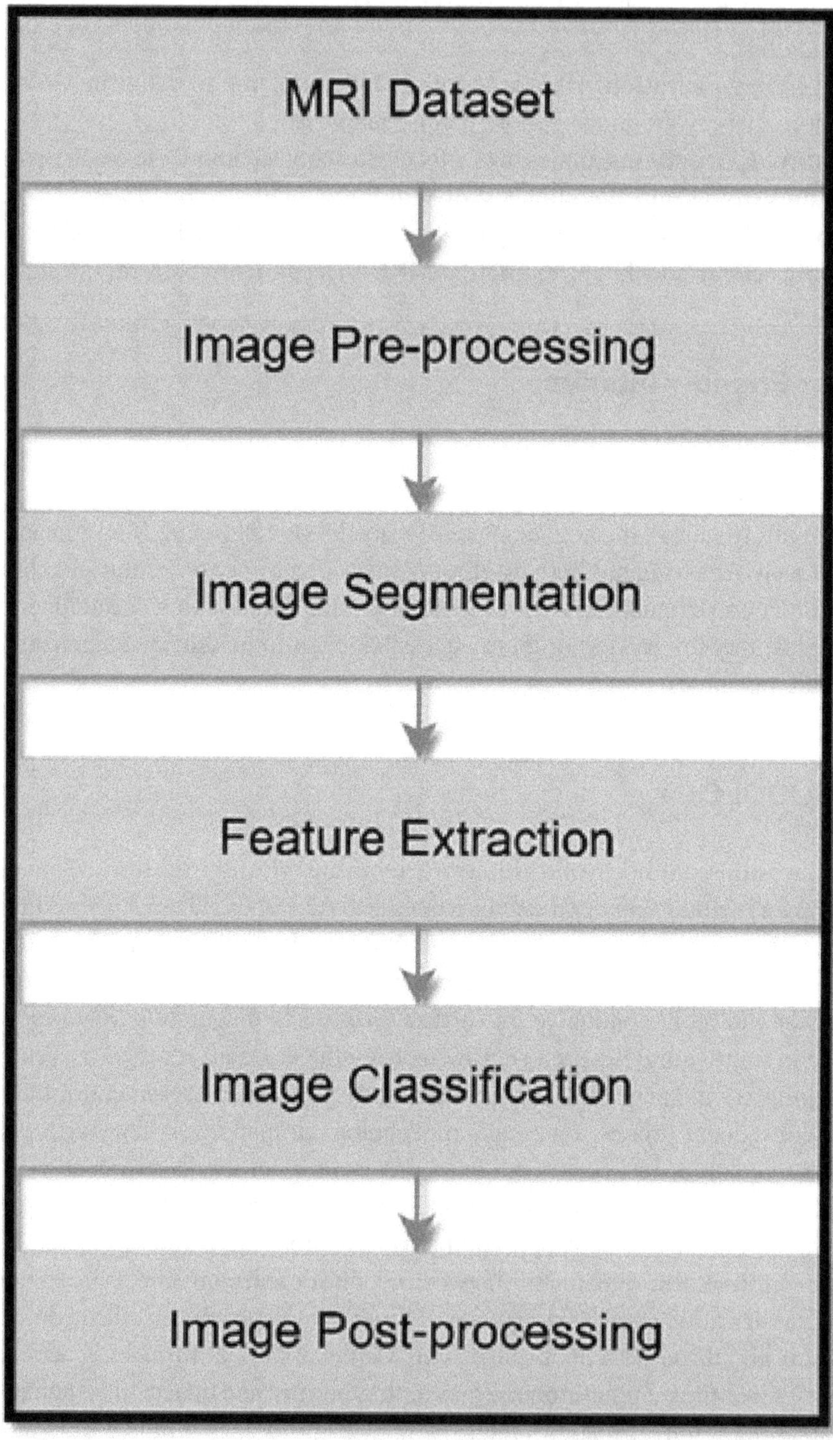

Step 1: Image Pre-Processing

First, the image enhancement is the process connected with a set of image processing methods for improving the quality of medical images to improve their visibility in connection to the brain tumor. Some enhancement methods for preprocessing MRI images can be performed, such as Gaussian filtering, contrast stretching, or histogram equalization, among others.

For example, let's say we have an image.

- Load an MRI image and convert it to grayscale.
- Median filtering is a noise reduction technique that suppresses the noise in the image and then enhances the contrast of the image.
- CLAHE (Contrast Limited Adaptive Histogram Equalization) technique allows improving the image. CLAHE is considered to be one of the best algorithms for image enhancement, since it adapts the contrast to local regions of the image, enhancing the contrast of the brain tumor region while retaining the contrasts within the surrounding healthy tissues.

Alternatively, an algorithm for CL:

- The image can be broken into small regions, forming tiles.
- Apply histogram equalization to each tile for contrast enhancement.
- Limiting the amplification of contrast in each tile so that the amplified noise is not further increased (Kabir, 2020).

Step 2: Image Segmentation

The most popular method of segmentation is the simplest method of "Global Thresholding", which assumes that there is some threshold value that can separate foreground and background pixel intensities. From this, we can calculate the threshold value by using the histogram of the image that gives information on pixel intensity distribution. All the pixels below the threshold that are in the gray image are taken into the background. Meanwhile, all the foreground pixels are above the threshold according to how the global threshold was set (Ayadi et al., 2021).

Elaborate steps for the global thresholding segmentation:

- Take the given input image and convert it into grayscale.
- Compute the histogram of the grayscale image.
- Derive the Cumulative Distribution Function (or CDF) from the histogram.
- Normalize the CDF values between 0 and 1.

- Choosing a threshold value may be based on one of the criteria to be achieved, for instance, when to maximize the intra-class variance or limit the inter-class variance.
- Set the intensity values larger than the threshold to 1 (foreground) and smaller than the threshold to 0 (background) to threshold the image.

Step 3: Feature Extraction

Finding and extracting pertinent characteristics from a picture that can be utilized for additional analysis and classification is a crucial stage in the process of feature extraction. CNN can be employed for feature extraction utilizing the windowing technique in the case of brain tumor identification. The process involves subdividing the picture into small sub-images or windows, then applying CNN to each window to extract important features.

Windowing is a technique in medicine that serves to assist in the mapping of values for contrast and brightness improvement from one group of values of pixels to a new range of values. Both these happen together: a pixel value window is selected in a certain range, and then it is scaled to the whole range of pixel intensity values. This helps accentuate the detailed salient features presented in the image, hence making them visible to the human eye.

Specifically, it is used to denote the input image by I (x, y). On the other hand, the windowed output image is denoted by I_w.

The windowing function can thus be described as follows:

$$I\_w (x, y) = (I (x, y) - L) * (H - L) / (H - L)$$

where H represents the window's top limit and L its lower limit. This function scales the pixel values within the window to the full range of intensity values.

Step 4: Image Classification

The classification of images involves attributing labels or categories based on their visual properties. In the realm of detecting brain tumors, features derived from images through Convolutional Neural Networks (CNNs) play a pivotal role in discerning whether an image harbors a tumor. Diverse algorithms like Support Vector Machines (SVM), Random Forests, and k-Nearest Neighbors (k-NN) classifiers can be harnessed for the purpose of image categorization. The efficacy of a brain tumor detection system heavily relies on the judicious selection of classification techniques and specific parameters. Consequently, it becomes indispensable to meticulously scrutinize and juxtapose different methodologies to identify the most pertinent one for the given scenario.

CNNs have garnered considerable acclaim owing to their adeptness in distilling intricate details from images, rendering them well-suited for tasks entailing image classification. These neural networks exhibit formidable capabilities, yielding highly precise models in applications related to image categorization, particularly when trained on copious datasets. In essence, the triumph of a brain tumor detection system hinges upon the deployment of apt image classification methodologies and algorithms. A thorough assessment and juxtaposition of myriad approaches are imperative to ascertain optimal efficacy and precision in discerning tumors from medical images. By harnessing the prowess of CNNs and other sophisticated algorithms, healthcare practitioners can augment the effectiveness of brain tumor detection and diagnosis, thereby ultimately ameliorating patient care and outcomes.

Step 5: Convolutional Neural Network

One of the main approaches of deep learning, which found great application in the area of images processing, including tasks like recognition, segmentation, and classification, is a convolutional neural network (CNN). It is a network of so many layers of nodes that process the incoming visual data convolutionally in order to extract patterns and features that can be applied to classification. For example, in the context of image segmentation with the target to detect brain tumors from magnetic resonance images, the training of CNNs is the process to prepare the model for processing MRI images by defining areas of images indicating a presence of a tumor.

The convolutional layer is the first layer of a convolutional network. While convolutional layers can be followed by additional convolutional layers or pooling layers, the fully-connected layer is the final layer. With each layer, the CNN increases in its complexity, identifying greater portions of the image. Earlier layers focus on simple features, such as colors and edges. As the image data progresses through the layers of the CNN, it starts to recognize larger elements or shapes of the object until it finally identifies the intended object.

A CNN would take MRI images as input and, after a few convolutional layers, would give an output probability map for the existence of the tumor throughout all the regions of an image. It can then be used to segment a tumor and make a diagnosis. In this context, a CNN convolutional layer in the context of detecting brain tumors from MRI segmentation involves applying a series of filters to the input MRI image in order to extract some relevant features. These filters are also called kernels and are slid over the image to compute the dot product in a local region between the filter weights and the image pixels.

They are usually small in size, like, say, 3x3 or 5x5. This process is repeated many times to build a feature map, which indicates highlight patterns or structures in the image. These feature maps are then processed by additional layers, like pooling layers, or more convolutional layers in order to down-sample further or to extract higher-level features. After passing the output of CNN through, it is finally put into a fully connected layer or SoftMax layer where it generates the final prediction. In more layman terms, these layers of CNN would be trained on the fundamental comprehension of texture, shape, or even intensity changes in tissues that could hint at the presence of tumors. The CNN can learn to recognize such patterns and hence apply it to the new images by training it exhaustively on a huge dataset of MRI images with or without tumors. An important note that a CNN's architecture and the corresponding hyperparameters, like the number and size of layers, filters, and learning rate, are significantly important toward good performance on this task. Therefore, network design and tuning should be done carefully in order to bring out the best results.

Step 6: Image Post Processing

To be able to find out the tumor portion in the brain, clarity pictures were post-processed using morphological operations. Erosion and dilation are the morphological operations, through which noise can be removed and gaps can be filled in the image. An erosion reduces the sizes of the objects in the image, while dilation enlarges the objects. In this work, they are applied with an operation structuring element that defines the shape and size of the neighborhood to be considered.

If we consider two sets: set A to represent the image and set B to be the structural element, then the dilatation of A by B is defined as follows:

I wrote it exactly as the teacher has told me. Similarly, A's erosion by B is defined as follows:

$(A \ominus B)(x, y) = \min \{$

Where (i, j) is a location in the structuring element and (x, y) is its center.

Step 7: Dataset Size and Diversity

The dataset used consists of MRI scans. The dataset contained nearly 3000 MRI scans, out of which 1500 are those affected by a tumor and 1500 of a normal brain. The MRI scans dataset has been adopted from various origins over the internet. Eighty percent of the data are used for training the model, and about twenty percent is tested.

Total no. of images used -> 3000
Images with tumors: Yes

Tumor-free images [No] – 15080-20 Training-Testing is employed, where 20% of the data is utilized for model testing, whereas the remaining 80% of the data is used to train the model.

Step 8: Proposed System

The processing of a brain tumor detection and classification image proposed system is done by using a pipeline image processing technique. The methods included in this were tumor segmentation using global threshold segmentation, image classification using morphological operations and windowing techniques, preprocessing of the image using Contrast Limited Adaptive Histogram Equalization (CLAHE), and a Convolutional Neural Network (CNN) algorithm to classify its type. A user interface has been made using React.js and Flask to develop an interface through which users will upload their MRI images and get predictive output for the detection of a brain tumor and its classification. The system should deliver reliable and accurate results to health providers in a very easy, reliable, and timely manner.

The proposed mechanism for brain tumor identification and categorization employs an elaborate image processing pipeline methodology. This methodology incorporates diverse techniques to ensure precise and dependable outcomes. Primarily, tumor segmentation is executed using a global threshold segmentation strategy. This strategy effectively segregates the tumor area from the neighboring brain tissues, laying a solid foundation for subsequent scrutiny. Subsequently, image classification is conducted through the application of morphological operations and windowing techniques. These operations refine the segmented images, heightening the accuracy of tumor classification. Moreover, preprocessing of the images is conducted using Contrast Limited Adaptive Histogram Equalization (CLAHE). This preprocessing maneuver enhances image quality, facilitating the detection of subtle tumor irregularities.

Furthermore, a Convolutional Neural Network (CNN) algorithm is employed to categorize the tumor type. CNNs are renowned for their proficiency in extracting intricate features from images, thereby enabling precise classification of tumor varieties. To streamline user interaction, a user interface has been developed utilizing React.js and Flask. This interface enables users to effortlessly upload MRI images and receive predictive outputs for tumor identification and classification. By furnishing a user-friendly interface, the system ensures accessibility and simplicity for healthcare practitioners.

In summary, the system endeavors to furnish healthcare practitioners with dependable and precise outcomes in a timely manner. By harnessing advanced image processing methodologies and machine learning algorithms, it facilitates efficient identification and classification of brain tumors, thereby contributing to enhanced patient care and outcomes.

RESULTS AND DISCUSSION

Figure 2 displays and MRI image and the image has been processed and analyzed using the proposed system's pipeline of image processing techniques.

Figure 2. Output of Visualization

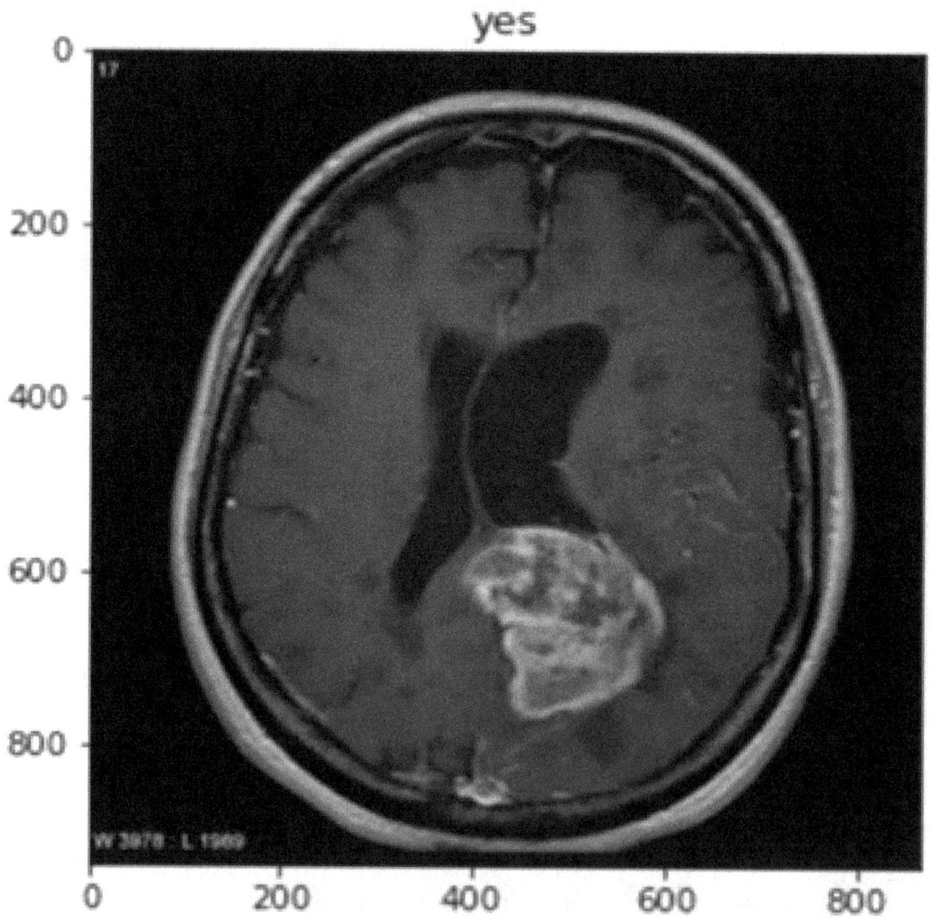

Figure 3 depicts multiple MRI images of brain tumors arranged within a single frame. Each image represents a different case or instance of brain tumor detection.

Figure 3. MRI Images of Brain Tumors

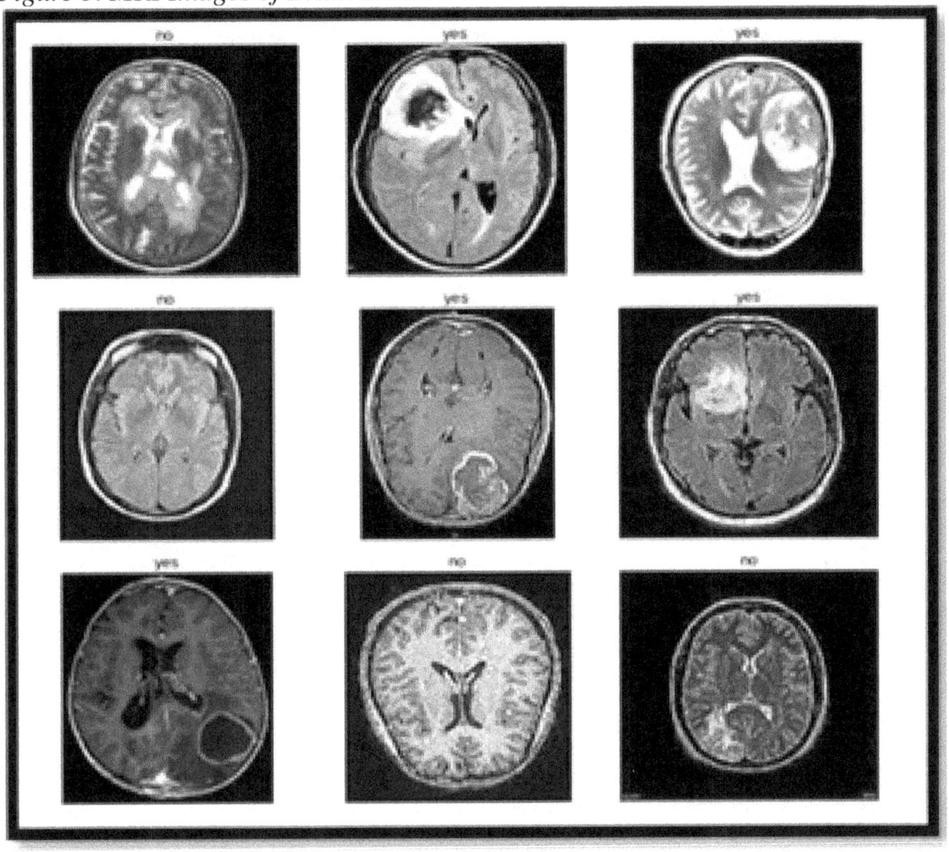

Performance Evaluation

- **Accuracy: 0.98**

Figure 4 graph shows the accuracy of the Convolutional Neural Network (CNN) algorithm used for brain tumor classification against the number of epochs during training.

Figure 4. Accuracy vs EPOC

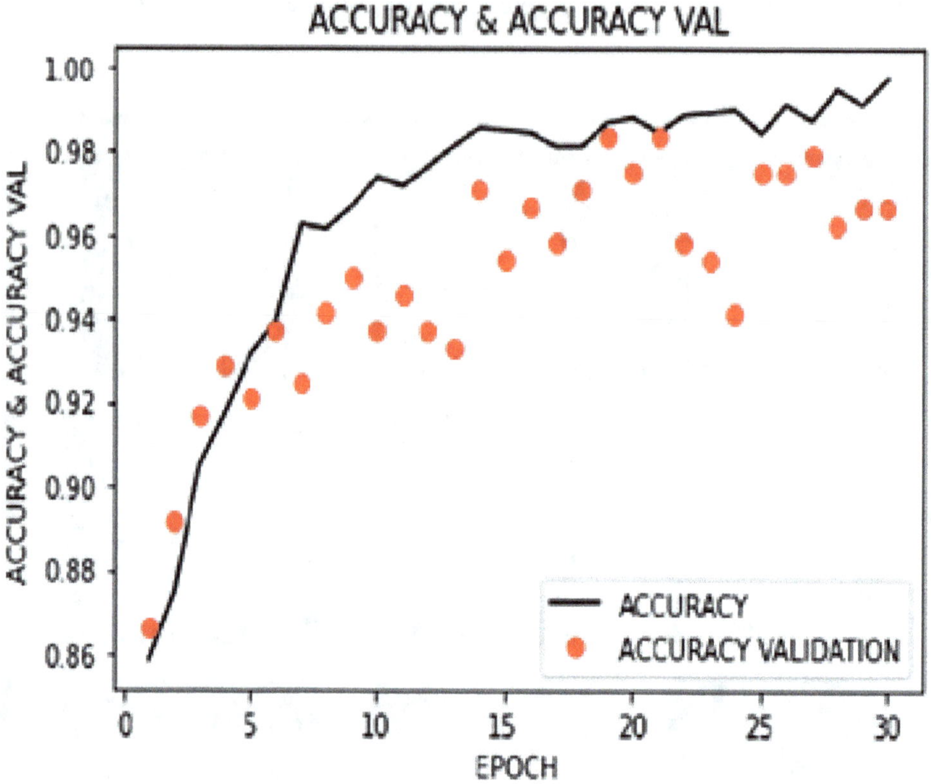

Figure 5 graph illustrates the loss function's value of the Convolutional Neural Network (CNN) model over training epochs.

Figure 5. Loss and EPOC

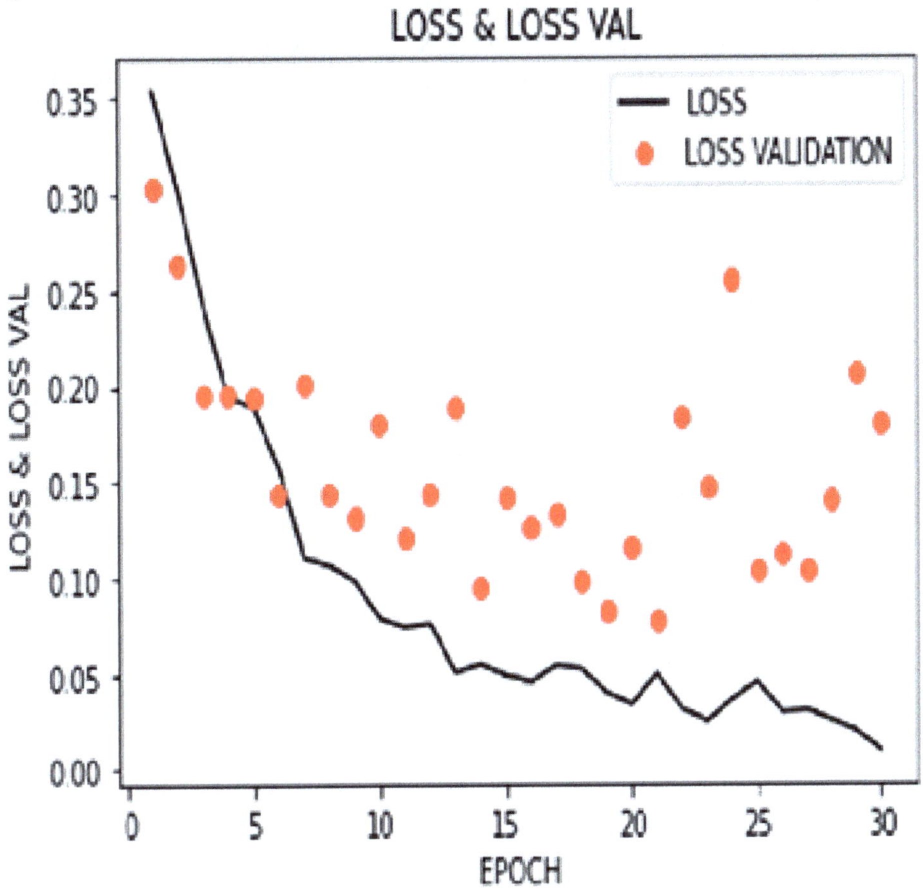

APPLICATIONS

- Augmented Diagnostic Precision: Deep learning constructs, particularly Convolutional Neural Networks (CNNs), exhibit prodigious potential in refining the precision of brain tumor identification via MRI scans. These algorithms can discern and categorize tumors with exceptional accuracy, enabling early detection essential for efficacious treatment and enhanced patient prognoses.
- Automated Delineation: Employing CNNs for the automatic segmentation of MRI imagery streamlines the diagnostic workflow by reducing the necessity

for manual analysis by radiologists. This mechanization expedites diagnosis and diminishes the burden on healthcare practitioners.

- Enhanced Visual Clarity: Methods such as Contrast Limited Adaptive Histogram Equalization (CLAHE) markedly augment the perceptibility of brain tumors in MRI scans. By augmenting the lucidity of these images, CLAHE assists in the detection of anomalies, especially in instances where tumors are inconspicuous or situated in difficult-to-visualize regions.
- Intuitive Interfaces: The integration of deep learning models into intuitive interfaces allows healthcare providers to seamlessly upload MRI images and receive prognostic outputs. This democratization of access to sophisticated diagnostic tools extends their reach to a broader spectrum of healthcare institutions, including those with constrained resources.
- Tailored Therapeutic Strategies: By meticulously identifying and categorizing brain tumors, deep learning models facilitate the formulation of bespoke treatment regimens. This process encompasses selecting the most appropriate therapeutic modality—be it surgery, radiotherapy, or chemotherapy—tailored to the specific type and characteristics of the tumor.
- Ongoing Surveillance: Deep learning models can be harnessed for the continuous surveillance of brain tumor progression through periodic MRI scans. This capability is vital for evaluating treatment efficacy and implementing timely modifications to the therapeutic plan as necessary.

CHALLENGES

- Data Integrity and Abundance: The efficacy of deep learning constructs is profoundly contingent on the integrity and volume of the training data. MRI datasets must be extensive and heterogeneous to encapsulate the variability in tumor morphology across diverse patients. Procuring such all-encompassing datasets poses a formidable challenge.
- Computational Demand: The training and deployment of deep learning models necessitate substantial computational prowess, particularly potent GPUs. This requirement can pose a considerable impediment for smaller medical facilities or those operating in resource-limited environments.
- Model Interpretability: Deep learning models, especially profound CNNs, frequently function as enigmatic entities, rendering it arduous to elucidate the basis of their specific prognostications. This opacity can be problematic for clinicians who require comprehension of the underlying rationale of a diagnosis.

- Seamless Workflow Integration: The incorporation of deep learning models into pre-existing clinical workflows is intricate. It demands compatibility with hospital information systems, adherence to data privacy and security protocols, and comprehensive training for personnel to adeptly utilize the new technologies.
- Regulatory Compliance: Medical apparatuses and diagnostic instruments predicated on deep learning models must undergo exhaustive evaluation and secure regulatory endorsements prior to clinical deployment. This process is often protracted and financially burdensome.
- Generalization Across Varied Demographics: Deep learning models trained on specific datasets may exhibit limited generalizability across diverse demographics with differing characteristics or MRI scanning methodologies. Ensuring robustness and adaptability across varied patient cohorts is a significant hurdle.
- Ethical and Juridical Considerations: The employment of AI in healthcare invokes ethical and juridical deliberations, encompassing concerns regarding patient consent, data proprietorship, and the potential for algorithmic bias. Addressing these issues is imperative to ensure the ethical application of deep learning in medical diagnostics.

CONCLUSION

This study has demonstrated the potential of deep learning, specifically Convolutional Neural Networks (CNNs), in revolutionizing brain tumor detection through MRI segmentation. By leveraging the unique intensity variations in MRI images caused by the high-water concentration and abundance of hydrogen atoms in tumor areas, our methodology achieves a remarkable 98% accuracy in brain tumor detection. The integration of the Contrast Limited Adaptive Histogram Equalization (CLAHE) algorithm for optimal contrast enhancement further underscores the efficacy of our approach.

Moreover, this research aligns with the Sustainable Development Goals (SDGs) by promoting health and well-being (SDG 3) through advanced diagnostic technologies. It highlights the importance of resilient healthcare systems capable of withstanding climate change impacts, ensuring continuous and equitable access to brain tumor detection and treatment services. By integrating deep learning and robust imaging techniques, we contribute to building resilient communities that can better respond to health challenges posed by environmental changes.

Future research should expand to include a comprehensive database of information on all types of brain tumors, providing a broader range of precautions and treatment options. Implementing machine learning algorithms to recommend the best treatment centers based on individual patient preferences and proximity can enhance patient care. Secure and efficient data management systems are also crucial for easy retrieval and updating of patient information, incorporating data from various sources, and using analytics to monitor progress and treatment effectiveness.

FUTURE SCOPE

There are several future directions that can be explored based on the proposed features for the website's user interface. Future research can focus on integrating more comprehensive information on brain tumor types, including a wider range of precautions and treatment options for each type. In terms of suggesting the best treatment center for brain tumor patients, future research can explore the use of machine learning algorithms to personalize recommendations based on individual patient needs, such as proximity to their location and treatment preferences. This can also involve leveraging patient data to better understand the effectiveness of different treatments and the factors that contribute to positive outcomes.

Finally, in terms of keeping patient records, future research can focus on developing secure and effective data management systems that allow doctors to easily access and update patient information. This can involve integrating patient data from multiple sources and leveraging analytics tools to track patient progress and treatment effectiveness. Overall, these future directions can lead to more accurate diagnosis, personalized treatment options, and improved patient outcomes for those with brain tumors.

REFERENCES

Ahmed, N., & Sabir, M. (2015). A superior achievement of brain tumor detection using segmentation based on F-transform. In *2015 IEEE International Conference*. IEEE.

Al-Galal, S. A. Y., Alshaikhli, I. F. T., & Abdulrazzaq, M. M. (2021). MRI brain tumor medical images analysis using deep learning techniques: A systematic review. *Health and Technology*, *11*(2), 267–282. DOI: 10.1007/s12553-020-00514-6

Ali, M., Gilani, S. O., Waris, A., Zafar, K., & Jamil, M. (2020). Brain tumour image segmentation using deep networks. *IEEE Access : Practical Innovations, Open Solutions*, *8*, 153589–153598. DOI: 10.1109/ACCESS.2020.3018160

Ayadi, W., Elhamzi, W., Charfi, I., & Atri, M. (2021). Deep CNN for brain tumor classification. *Neural Processing Letters*, *53*(1), 671–700. DOI: 10.1007/s11063-020-10398-2

Chandra, S. K., & Bajpai, M. K. (2018). Effective algorithm for benign brain tumor detection using fractional calculus. In Proceedings of TENCON 2018 - 2018 IEEE Region 10 Conference. IEEE.

Dhanve, V., & Kumar, M. (2017). Detection of brain tumor using k-means segmentation based on object labeling algorithm. In *2017 IEEE International Conference on Power, Control, Signals and Instrumentation Engineering (ICPCSI)*. IEEE.

Ezhilarasi, R., & Varalakshmi, P. (2018). Tumor detection in the brain using faster R-CNN. In 2018 2nd International Conference on I-SMAC (IoT in Social, Mobile, Analytics and Cloud) (I-SMAC) (pp. 388–392). IEEE. https://doi.org/DOI: 10.1109/I-SMAC.2018.8653736

Gobhinath, S., Anandkumar, S., Dhayalan, R., Ezhilbharathi, P., & Haridharan, R. (2021). Human brain tumor detection and classification by medical image processing. In 2021 7th International Conference on Advanced Computing and Communication Systems (ICACCS). IEEE. https://doi.org/DOI: 10.1109/ICACCS51430.2021.9441877

Hebli, A., & Gupta, S. (2017). Brain tumor prediction and classification using support vector machine. In *2017 IEEE International Conference on Advances in Computing, Communications and Informatics (ICACCI)*. IEEE.

Kabir, M. A. (2020). Early-stage brain tumor detection on MRI image using a hybrid technique. In 2020 IEEE Region 10 Symposium (TENSYMP). IEEE.

Kaur, N., & Sharma, M. (2017). Brain tumor detection using self-adaptive K-means clustering. In *2017 International Conference on Energy, Communication, Data Analytics and Soft Computing (ICECDS)*. IEEE.

Kumar, S., Dhir, R., & Chaurasia, N. (2021). Brain tumor detection analysis using CNN: A review. In *2021 International Conference on Artificial Intelligence and Smart Systems (ICAIS)* (pp. 1061–1067). IEEE. https://doi.org/DOI: 10.1109/ICAIS50930.2021.9395920

Rahman, M. L., Reza, A. W., & Shabuj, S. I. (2022). An internet of things-based automatic brain tumor detection system. *Indonesian Journal of Electrical Engineering and Computer Science*, *25*(1), 214–222. DOI: 10.11591/ijeecs.v25.i1.pp214-222

Swami, M., & Verma, D. (2020). An algorithmic detection of brain tumor using image filtering and segmentation of various radiographs. In 2020 7th International Conference on Signal Processing and Integrated Networks (SPIN). IEEE.

Vaishnavee, K. B., & Amshakala, K. (2015). An automated MRI brain image segmentation and tumor detection using SOM-clustering and proximal support vector machine classifier. In *2015 IEEE International Conference on Engineering and Technology (ICETECH)*. IEEE.

Yang, T., & Song, J. (2018). An automatic brain tumor image segmentation method based on the U-net. In 2018 IEEE 4th International Conference on Computer and Communications (ICCC) (pp. 1600–1604). IEEE.

Chapter 5
AI in Managing Chronic Diseases

Priti Mangesh Bharambe
https://orcid.org/0009-0000-8700-9822
MIT Arts, Commerce, and Science College, India

Santosh Jagtap
MIT Arts, Commerce, and Science College, India

ABSTRACT

Chronic diseases, including diabetes, cardiovascular disorders, and cancer, are responsible for more than 70% of deaths worldwide, placing considerable pressure on healthcare systems. This chapter explores the revolutionary impact of artificial intelligence in the management of chronic illnesses. By utilizing machine learning, AI can predict disease progression and offer highly accurate personalized treatment options. It enhances diagnostic processes, supports remote patient monitoring through wearable technology, and allows for real-time management of treatments, thereby improving patient outcomes. Significant topics covered include AI applications for the early detection of diabetic retinopathy and cancer, customized treatment plans, and automated medication management. Additionally, AI improves telemedicine by facilitating at-home monitoring of chronic conditions through the collection of real-time data. The chapter also addresses challenges such as data privacy and biases in AI, highlighting the importance of ethical considerations.

DOI: 10.4018/979-8-3373-0179-2.ch005

t © 2026, IGI Global Scientific Publishing. Copying or distributing in print or electronic forms without written permission of IGI Global Scientific Publishing is prohibited. Use of this chapter to enerative artificial intelligence (AI) technologies is expressly prohibited. The publisher reserves all rights to license its use for generative AI training and machine learning model development.

1. INTRODUCTION TO CHRONIC DISEASES AND HEALTHCARE CHALLENGES

1.1 Overview of Chronic Diseases

Overview of Chronic Diseases Long lasting health conditions that take time to develop and need ongoing medical attention or significantly limit activities of daily living are referred to as chronic diseases or non-communicable diseases (NCDs) (Collins & Varmus, 2015; Ashley, 2016). Common chronic diseases include:

- Diabetes: A disorder of metabolism that results in an elevated blood glucose level, if untreated, can cause extreme complications including kidney disease, loss of vision, neuropathy and cardiovascular disease. Both Type 1 and Type 2 diabetes are prevalent, and they are the leading contributors to the world's healthcare burden (Rajkomar et al., 2019; Miotto et al., 2018).
- Cardiovascular Disease (CVD): CVD – or conditions affecting the heart and blood vessels – includes coronary artery disease, hypertension, stroke, and heart failure. High rates of CVD, which remains a major cause of death worldwide, are largely attributable to risk factors, including hypertension, smoking and sedentary lifestyles (Topol, 2019; Bodenheimer & Sinsky, 2014).
- Cancer: Unless it becomes cancer, it's normally just a supercell that grows out of control. High morbidity and mortality rates are associated with common cancers, which include lung, breast, colorectal and prostate cancers. Treatment is often complex and expensive, and comes at a high cost to patients, and to healthcare systems (Esteva et al., 2017; Hood & Friend, 2011).

Figure 1. Chronic Diseases Complications Diagram

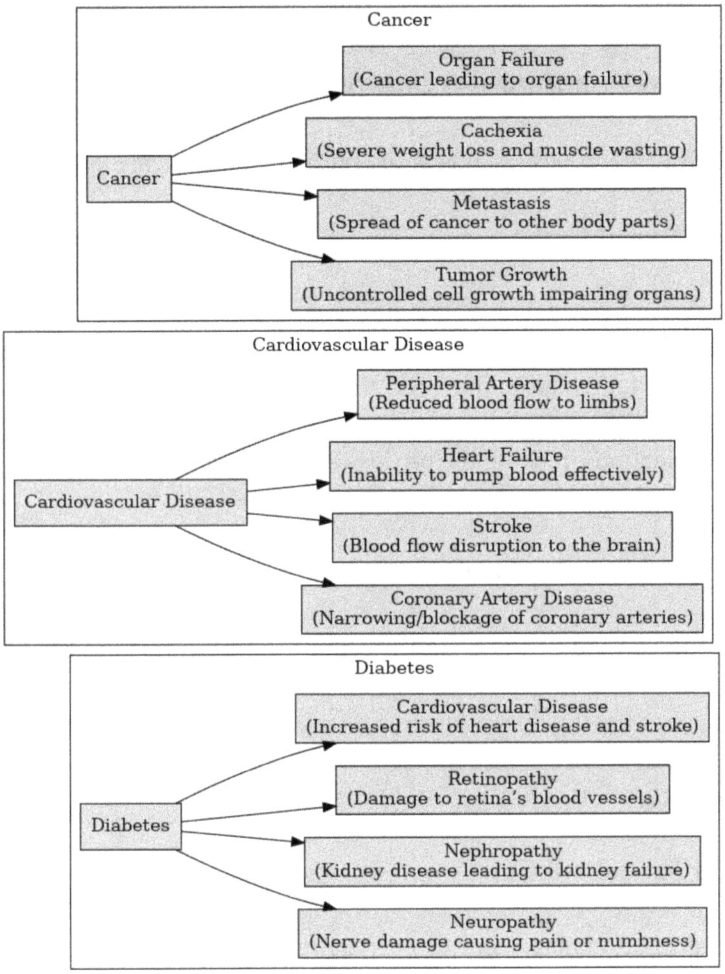

These are common chronic conditions with which we are all familiar, these chronic conditions rely on your lifestyle, genetics, and your environment. In general, they're generally incurable, but they're also possible to manage and with treatment, patients can often maintain a high quality of life (Ashley, 2016; Collins & Varmus, 2015).

AI applications in the management of chronic diseases encompass a diverse array of functions, such as early diagnosis, personalized treatment, continuous monitoring, and ensuring medication compliance. These innovations have significantly transformed conventional methods by utilizing machine learning to detect patterns, forecast risks, and suggest interventions customized to the specific requirements of each patient. This chapter delves into these topics comprehensively, emphasizing the transformative influence of AI on healthcare systems worldwide (Rajkomar et al., 2019; Miotto et al., 2018, Topol, 2019; Morley et al., 2020).

1.2 Impact on Healthcare Systems

Chronic diseases impose a substantial burden on healthcare systems due to:

1. **High Treatment Costs:**

Chronic disease management requires continual management, ongoing monitoring, medications, and complex interventions (Bodenheimer & Sinsky, 2014). To manage diabetes, for instance, one takes daily medication, frequently checks blood sugar levels, and consults healthcare professionals through periodic health checkups to avoid complications, making the process a heavy load on healthcare expenditure (Collins & Varmus, 2015).

2. **Increased Hospitalization Rates:**

People with chronic diseases are more likely to need frequent hospitalizations and readmissions (Bodenheimer & Sinsky, 2014). Repeated hospital stays due to conditions such as heart failure, diabetic foot ulcers, and other diabetes-related complications including retinopathy place strain on hospital capacities and significantly increase healthcare costs (Ashley, 2016).

3. **Need for Specialized Care:**

Chronic disease management often requires specialized healthcare providers such as endocrinologists, cardiologists, and oncologists (Ashley, 2016). The cost of such specialized care is high and its availability is often limited to urban centers, which widens the gap in access to quality healthcare among rural and underserved communities (Collins & Varmus, 2015).

4. **Resource Allocation and Workforce Demand:**

Resources required for the treatment of chronic diseases are substantial in terms of both medical supplies and trained healthcare professionals (Bashshur et al., 2014). Chronic diseases account for an increasing proportion of global morbidity and mortality, placing sustained pressure on healthcare systems and affecting their ability to deliver high-quality care due to workforce shortages and limited resource availability (Bodenheimer & Sinsky, 2014).

5. **Long-Term Dependency on Healthcare Services:**

Unlike acute diseases, chronic diseases require healthcare services over extended periods, often spanning many years (Hood & Friend, 2011). This long-term dependency presents challenges for healthcare systems in maintaining consistent and effective care while balancing resource allocation for other healthcare needs (Morley et al., 2020).

Figure 2. Cause and effect diagram

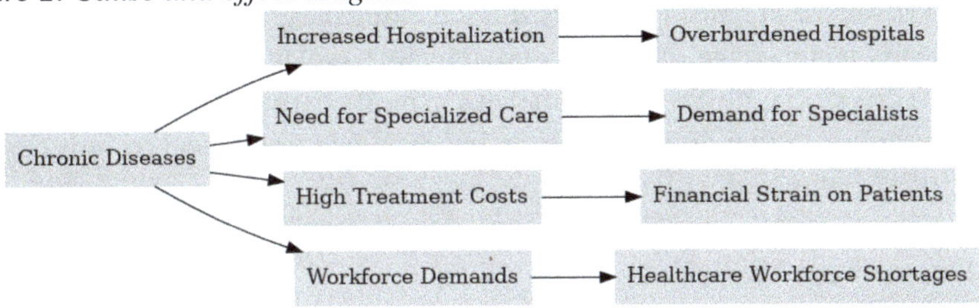

Figure 3. Global Healthcare Cost Attributes

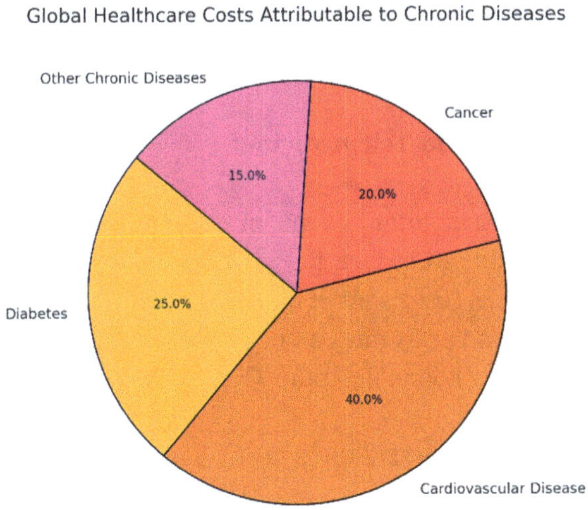

1.3 Need for Innovative Solutions

The challenges posed by chronic diseases require an innovation in healthcare delivery that offers to reduce costs, improve patient outcomes and offer innovative approaches that will address the challenges of healthcare delivery (Topol, 2019; Rajkomar et al., 2019). Key areas for innovation include:

- **Early Diagnosis and Prevention:**

Using advanced diagnostic devices and screening programmes to detect chronic diseases early and manage risk factors proactively (Ashley, 2016). Other examples include AI driven diagnostic algorithm that can notify early signs of the disease like cancer or cardiovascular abnormalities in imaging data or medical records (Esteva et al., 2017; Miotto et al., 2018).

- **Personalized Medicine:**

Using predictive analytics and targeting treatment based on individual patient profiles (Collins & Varmus, 2015). This streamlines intervention because it diminishes the possibility that interventions will lead to adverse effects and be better at achieving the overall outcomes (Hood & Friend, 2011). Personalized treatment plans can be created with AI that will analyze a patient's genetic data, lifestyle and medical history (Rajkomar et al., 2019; Topol, 2019).

- **Remote Monitoring and Telemedicine:**

By using technology to monitor patients in real time, including through remote consultations, it is possible to reduce the number of hospital visits in particular for patients in remote areas (Bashshur et al., 2014). Vital health metrics like blood pressure, glucose levels and heart rate can be tracked by wearable devices and then acted upon to prevent early hospitalizations (Keesara et al., 2020).

- **AI in Predictive Analytics:**

By using AI algorithms, healthcare providers can evaluate patients at increased risk of complications or readmission to the hospital and reallocate resources accordingly and prevent and stay ahead of adverse outcomes (Rajkomar et al., 2019; Miotto et al., 2018).

- **Automated Systems for Medication and Lifestyle Management:**

Using AI, these systems can also help support medication adherence, remind patients to make lifestyle modifications, and monitor that compliance (Morley et al., 2020). In particular, lifestyle (including diet and physical activity) based recommendations have powerful potential to be automated, especially in the form of reminders (Bodenheimer & Sinsky, 2014).

Figure 4. AI Applications in Chronic Disease Management and Their Feedback Loop for Improved Patient Outcomes.

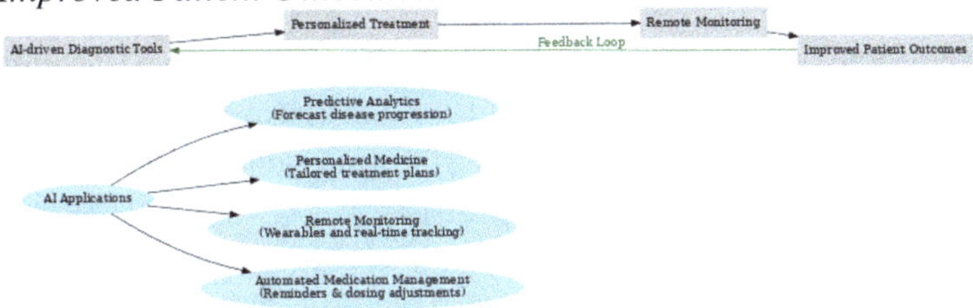

These innovative solutions can address those chronic diseases and ease the pressures on the healthcare system, improve patient quality of life, and lay the foundation for a more sustainable, efficient healthcare model of the future.

Figure 5. AI-Driven Process for Enhancing Patient Quality of Life through Diagnostics, Treatment, and Monitoring.

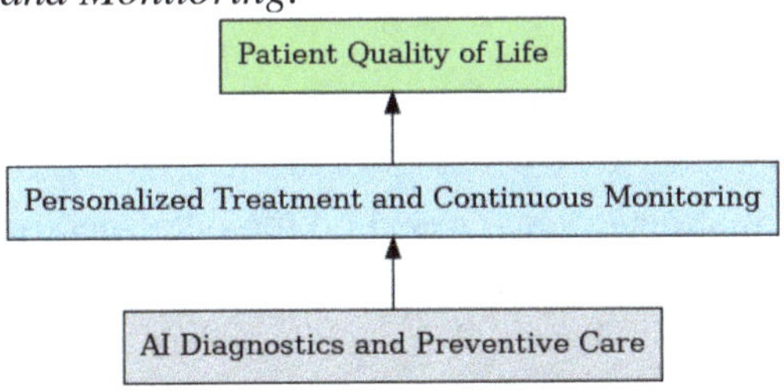

2. CHRONIC DISEASE MANAGEMENT WITH THE ROLE OF AI

Using Artificial Intelligence (AI) for the management of chronic disease is transforming how diseases are detected, how treatments are tailored, how medications can be best adhered to, and how patients can be most effectively monitored. It helps chronic diseases, which are often long term and complex, as they benefit from the ability of AI to look at large datasets, find patterns, and make predictive assessments for healthcare providers. In this section, I take a peek into how AI applications are helping manage chronic diseases better and more effectively, and in turn, making it seamless for the healthcare ecosystem to function better Rajkomar et al. (2019); Topol (2019); Miotto et al. (2018).

2.1 AI in Chronic Disease Treatment and Management

2.1.1 Predictive Analytics and Early Detection

As with any other subject area, AI, especially through machine learning and deep learning models, makes it possible to detect chronic diseases early on by examining a host of variables including medical records, lab tests, genetic profiles, and imaging data Rajkomar et al. (2019); Miotto et al. (2018).

Example: More and more, in other words, AI is being used to identify early signs of diseases like diabetes and cardiovascular disease Topol (2019). For example, predictive models to predict the onset of Type 2 diabetes based on lifestyle factors and genetic data identify who needs preventive intervention before the disease manifests fully Collins & Varmus (2015); Ashley (2016).

Google DeepMind's algorithm, for example, has shown the capability to identify more than 50 vision-threatening eye diseases through retinal scans, achieving accuracy levels similar to those of expert ophthalmologists Rajkomar et al. (2019); Topol (2019). This advancement enables timely intervention for conditions such as diabetic retinopathy Topol (2019).

2.1.2 Personalized Treatment Plans

It can also tailor treatment plans, based on the data specific to each individual patient, namely genetics, lifestyle and medical history Ashley (2016); Collins & Varmus (2015). The ability to have this level of personalization improves treatment efficacy and decreases side effects by personalizing interventions to each patient's needs Topol (2019); Rajkomar et al. (2019).

Example: AI can also aid in finding the most effective drug combinations and doses for cancer patients, based on their tumor genetics and this information can help improve outcomes while lowering unnecessary side effects in treatment Hood & Friend (2011); Ashley (2016). AI driven decision support systems can suggest personalized lifestyle changes, exercise plans, dietary adjustments in cardiovascular diseases Topol (2019).

2.1.3 Medication Management and Adherence

Adherence to complex medication regimens is often difficult to manage for patients who have chronic diseases Bodenheimer & Sinsky (2014). Applications powered by AI monitor and support adherence with prescribed treatment Rajkomar et al. (2019).

Example: Patients can be reminded or notified by AI at a given time, adherence can be tracked using wearable devices, and AI can predict when a patient is going to miss a dose prompting timely interventions Miotto et al. (2018); Topol (2019).

2.1.4 Remote Monitoring and Patient Engagement

Real time monitoring is now possible with wearables and AI driven mobile applications that their provide listening to the patient's vital signs, symptoms, and adherence Topol (2019); Miotto et al. (2018). It gives room for early intervention if the patient's condition deteriorates, through this remote monitoring Keesara et al. (2020); Bashshur et al. (2014).

Example: Continuous glucose monitors that track a diabetic's glucose levels and send the data to their healthcare providers, or smart watches that monitor a patient's heart rate variability and inform a patient's healthcare providers, are examples of wearable devices. These metrics are analyzed by AI to find any strange patterns, such as strange glucose readings or an indication of close to heart failure and early action can be taken .

2.1.5 Enhanced Diagnostic Accuracy

AI enabled diagnostic tools can understand medical images, pathology slides, and patient data with high accuracy, at times equal to — or better than — the human eye Esteva et al. (2017); Rajkomar et al. (2019). The early detection of disease offered by AI driven diagnostics is key to effective chronic disease management Topol (2019).

Example: Images of retinas can be analyzed to detect presence of diabetic retinopathy (DR)— a complication of diabetes.The use of an AI driven approach means that blindness in diabetic patients is possible to detect early and lower the risk.

2.1.6 Telemedicine Support

Thanks to AI, telemedicine is changing, supporting healthcare providers with diagnostic assessment and therapy suggestions in the framework of virtual consultations Bashshur et al. (2014); Keesara et al. (2020). The use of telemedicine with

AI is a sure way to get patients with chronic diseases timely care, most especially those of the rural or underserved communities Bashshur et al. (2014).

Example: In remote healthcare, before a patient walks in the room, AI can scan them through symptoms and patient history, and suggest a diagnosis and suggestions, ideally leading to more informed and efficient care provided by the healthcare provider .

Table 1. AI Applications and Use Cases in Chronic Disease Management

AI Application	Use Case	Outcome
Predictive Analytics	Detecting risk of Type 2 diabetes progression	Early intervention and prevention
Diagnostics	Identifying diabetic retinopathy	Reduced risk of vision loss
Telemedicine	Remote monitoring for COPD patients	Reduced hospitalizations

2.2 How AI Supports Healthcare Systems in Addressing Chronic Disease Challenges

1. **Improving Healthcare Access:**

AI driven telemedicine platforms and remote monitoring tools enable patients in remote places to get access to high quality healthcare yet do not have to go to visit them very often Bashshur et al. (2014); Keesara et al. (2020). This is especially useful for patients who cannot move much or live an area where they don't have a lot of access healthcare facilities Bashshur et al. (2014).

2. **Reducing Healthcare Costs:**

AI helps to predict disease progression, improve patient medication adherence, and help identify early interventions to prevent costly complications and hospitalizations Rajkomar et al. (2019); Miotto et al. (2018). Not only is there less need for hospitalization, but remote monitoring using artificial intelligence alerts healthcare providers early and at the same time provides timely management of the symptoms Topol (2019).

3. **Addressing Workforce Shortages:**

Healthcare professionals can put trust in AI based automation to perform repetitive tasks, for instance, data entry and initial diagnostic assessments Bodenheimer

& Sinsky (2014). Thus, it encourages clinicians to spend less time on simpler cases, and help healthcare systems with more patients, with fewer resources Topol (2019).

4. **Ensuring Data-Driven Decision Making:**

With the use of AI to generate data based on patient history, real time data and predictive analytics, healthcare providers are given insight to help make informed decisions Rajkomar et al. (2019). They are invaluable in managing complex chronic diseases at which treatment requires continuous adjustment Miotto et al. (2018).

5. **Reducing Human Error in Diagnosis and Treatment:**

As AI has the ability to interpret huge chunks of data accurately, healthcare providers can use it to prevent diagnostic and treatment errors Esteva et al. (2017); Rajkomar et al. (2019). Such accuracy is critical in chronic disease management where time and precision of interventions have profound impact on patient outcomes Topol (2019).

6. **Enhancing Patient Education and Engagement:**

This application is an AI driven application where the patients are being educated about their condition, options for the treatment, and necessary lifestyle ones Ashley (2016). As one keeps an eye on it, AI creates information that is accessible and personalized making it easier for patients to take an active role in their own health, in turn, crucial for chronic disease management Hood & Friend (2011).

Chronic disease management can be enabled through the use of AI which holds the capabilities to analyze data in real time which then enables it to provide real time insights and allows for personalized interventions Rajkomar et al. (2019); Topol (2019). A new proactive approach to healthcare systems based on the integration of AI in healthcare systems, which equips both patients and providers with the capability to more actively manage chronic disease and thereby ensuring better health outcomes and a more sustainable health system Morley et al. (2020).

3. PREDICTIVE ANALYTICS AND DISEASE PROGRESSION FORECASTING

In chronic disease management, predictive analytics and disease progression forecasting are important predictive techniques that assist healthcare providers to predict possible complications, plan outpatient treatment and manage patient care proactively. Machine learning algorithms allow the healthcare systems to analyze large quantities of patient data and find patterns, identify what may or may not happen in the future. It provides an earlier, personalized and therefore more effective intervention that is needed in chronic diseases developing and progressing over long periods.

Figure 6. Predictive Analytics Workflow in Chronic Disease Management

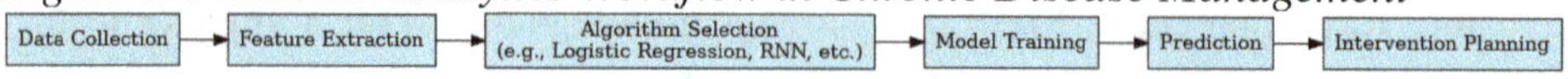

Machine Learning Algorithms for Predicting Disease Course and Outcomes

Figure 7. Hierarchical AI Models for Chronic Disease Management

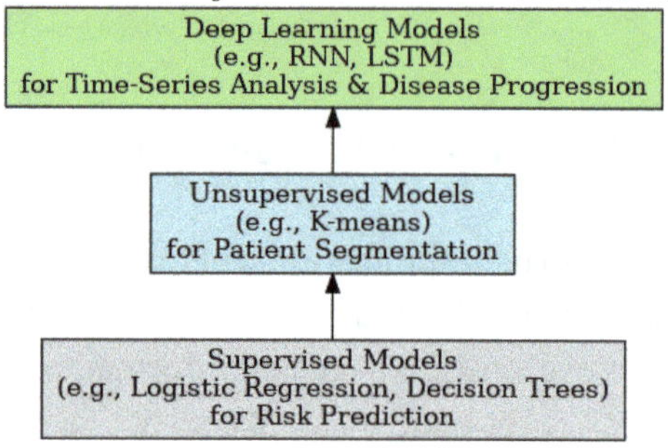

3.1 Machine Learning Model

1. **Supervised Learning Models:**

Like all algorithms, they learn from labeled data (data that has outcomes) to make predictions Rajkomar et al. (2019). Supervised learning models are utilized in chronic disease management in predicting disease onset, progression or the degree of risk of complication for a disease state Miotto et al. (2018).

Example: Predicting the onset of disease (e.g., transition from prediabetes to Type 2 diabetes) is usually done with logistic regression and decision trees. These models predict the likelihood of disease progression from risk factors such as age, BMI, family history and lifestyle .

2. **Unsupervised Learning Models:**

Detecting trends and clusters in unlabeled data (data with no predefined results) are what these algorithms pick up Miotto et al. (2018). Unsupervised models are useful in chronic disease management in segmenting patients based on their risk profile and can provide targeted intervention for patient groups Rajkomar et al. (2019).

Example: While there are many clustering algorithms such as the K means, these algorithms group diabetic patients based on factors such as glucose level, weight, activity level. Treatment plans for each group are individually elucidated within each cluster.

3. **Recurrent Neural Networks (RNNs) and Long Short-Term Memory Networks (LSTMs):**

These deep learning models are intended for time series data and are strongly applicable to prognostic of course of chronic diseases that steadily develop Miotto et al. (2018).

Example: Since long time series data on patient biomarkers such as kidney function, blood pressure, etc. can be used to predict the progression of chronic kidney disease (CKD) in an RNN or an LSTM way Rajkomar et al. (2019). For doctors, the model can predict the rate at which kidney function will decline, and will help them plan appropriate timeframes for future interventions Topol (2019).

4. **Random Forest and Gradient Boosting Models:**

Ensemble models are comprised of multiple decision trees that predict accurately and are most often applied in chronic disease management because they are robust and accurate Miotto et al. (2018).

Example: Predictive cardiovascular event is attempted by applying random forest models to risk factors like cholesterol levels, blood pressure, smoking habits and family history Lastly, these models are really good at estimating the likelihood of having a heart attack or stroke and can help predict preemptively whether you need to make lifestyle or medication changes.

5. **Survival Analysis Models:**

In chronic disease progression, where the goal may be to delay adverse outcomes, these models will predict the time until an event occurs Hood & Friend (2011).

Example: A prediction of survival rates for cancer patients is made as a function of factors such as tumor type, patient demographics and treatment history using Cox proportional hazards models . This provides clinicians an opportunity to understand prognosis and make informed treatment decisions.

3.2 Case Studies and Examples of Predictive Models in Chronic Disease Management

1. Diabetes Management and Complication Prevention:

Case Study: To predict complications in diabetic patients (such as diabetic retinopathy or neuropathy), a machine learning model was ran in a hospital. The model then found high risk patients early by analyzing blood glucose levels, HbA1c measurements, blood pressure, and lifestyle data for them. The clinicians, able to act sooner with personalized treatment plans, thus decreased the frequency by which severe complications occurred.

Impact: Thanks to this predictive model, the hospital reduced readmission rates and enhanced patient outcomes and showed the effectiveness of machine learning in proactive diabetes management.

2. Heart Disease and Cardiovascular Risk Prediction:

Case Study: A foundational dataset that to build predictive models estimating risk of heart disease came from one of the longest running cardiovascular study, The Framingham Heart Study. Researchers use supervised learning techniques to build models that predetermine event of a cardiovascular disease with risk factors of age, cholesterol, blood pressure and smoking history. Since then, these models have been adapted into risk-calculators that healthcare providers worldwide use.

Impact: Preventive cardiology has relied on the Framingham-based models to tell millions of patients what lifestyle changes, such as diet and exercise, and what preventive medications, like the ones used to treat high cholesterol, can help to reduce their chances of developing heart disease.

3. Chronic Kidney Disease (CKD) Progression Forecasting:

Case Study: An LSTM model was applied to predict progression of CKD in patients over time by a healthcare provider. Using data points such as serum creatinine, blood urea nitrogen, blood pressure and protein in the urine to predict when a patient's kidney function will deteriorate to a point where they need to go on dialysis, the model could do this. Such forecasting enabled providers to time interventions, adjust medications and sometimes avert the need for dialysis.

Impact: By extending the patient's kidney function this approach delayed the need for dialysis, reduced costs to the healthcare system, and improved patient's quality of life.

4. Cancer Recurrence Prediction:

Case Study: Predictive analytics were used in oncology to predict cancer recurrence after treatment of patients. For example, machine learning models track information such as tumor type, genetic markers, a history of treatment and patient demographics that predict the odds of cancer coming back. For example, these models are used to determine which women with breast cancer will derive the most benefit from more aggressive follow up treatment.

Impact: The ability to predict recurrence allows hospitals to help high risk patients after treatment survive, along with providing mental and emotional support for patients.

5. Chronic Obstructive Pulmonary Disease (COPD) Exacerbation Prediction:

Case Study: Predictive models are used to predict exacerbations, the sudden worsening of the symptoms that most commonly result in hospitalization, in COPD management. With the help of machine learning techniques applied to data collected using wearables that track respiratory rate, oxygen saturation and patients' own symptoms, a model is created that predicts with some degree of certainty when an exacerbation is likely to occur.

Impact: An early warning provides for patients and providers to take precautionary steps, such as adjusting medications or oxygen therapy before emergency hospital visits, and improved patient quality of life.

Table 2. A table or grid that lists specific diseases, the predictive model used, and the outcome.

Disease	Predictive Model	Outcome
Diabetes	Logistic Regression	Risk of developing diabetes complications
Cardiovascular Disease	Random Forest	Likelihood of a heart attack
Chronic Kidney Disease	LSTM	Projected kidney function decline
Cancer	Cox Proportional Hazards	Prediction of recurrence risk

3.3 Benefits of Predictive Analytics in Chronic Disease Management

- Proactive Care:

Using predictive analytics, the healthcare providers can go from reactive care to proactive management, where potential complications are detected and dealt with before they become acute Rajkomar et al. (2019); Topol (2019).

- **Personalized Interventions:**

Health care providers are better able to tailor interventions that are more likely to be effective if they understand each patient's unique risk profile Ashley (2016); Collins & Varmus (2015).

- **Resource Optimization:**

Healthcare systems can use predictive models to provide more efficient resource allocation—allocating attention and efforts to high risk patients who just need more intensive monitoring and care and less in general Bodenheimer & Sinsky (2014); Miotto et al. (2018).

- **Improved Patient Outcomes:**

An ability to early predict and then intervene quickly gives patients with chronic disease better health outcomes, less hospitalizations and enhanced quality of life Topol (2019); Rajkomar et al. (2019).

Transforming chronic disease management through predictive analytics and disease progression forecasting is possible Miotto et al. (2018). With more sophisticated machine learning algorithms and bigger datasets these models will continue to be an essential piece of enabling personalized, proactive, and effective chronic disease care Rajkomar et al. (2019); Morley et al. (2020).

4 PERSONALIZED TREATMENT PLANNING WITH AI

4.1 Creating Individualized Treatment Plans with AI

AI empowered personalized treatment planning is transforming chronic disease management by allowing tailored care for each patient. Traditional "one size fits all" treatments often do not suit people living with chronic disease. AI algorithms are able to analyze data down to the granular level and be able to create very individualized treatment plans that optimize medication, lifestyle recommendations and monitor for the best possible results for each patient. In addition to treating more accurately, this approach also increases patient outcomes and satisfaction dramatically.

Creating Individualized Treatment Plans with AI Driven Approaches AI systems pull data from a number of sources, including electronic health records (EHRs), genetic profiles, wearable devices and patient reported data. Fits-all" treatments often fail to address the unique needs and responses of individuals with chronic diseases. By analyzing data at a granular level, AI algorithms can develop highly individualized treatment plans that optimize medication, lifestyle recommendations, and monitoring to achieve the best possible outcomes for each patient. This approach not only improves treatment accuracy but also significantly enhances patient outcomes and satisfaction.

4.2 AI-Driven Approaches to Create Individualized Treatment Plans

AI-Driven Approaches to Create Individualized Treatment Plans

1. **Patient Data Collection and Integration:**

AI systems aggregate data from a variety of sources, including electronic health records (EHRs), genetic profiles, wearable devices, and patient-reported data Rajkomar et al. (2019); Miotto et al. (2018). This comprehensive data set forms the foundation for creating a tailored treatment plan Topol (2019).

Example: For diabetes management, an AI system can integrate glucose readings, insulin sensitivity, dietary habits, and physical activity levels to provide personalized recommendations for insulin dosage and diet adjustments.

2. **Risk Stratification and Predictive Modeling:**

AI models categorize patients based on risk factors and disease severity, using predictive analytics to forecast likely disease progression or potential complications Rajkomar et al. (2019); Miotto et al. (2018). This stratification allows for different intensities of treatment based on a patient's risk profile Topol (2019).

Example: In cardiovascular care, predictive models assess patients' risk of heart attacks or strokes, allowing clinicians to assign higher-risk patients to more intensive monitoring and intervention protocols.

3. **Genomic Data Analysis for Precision Medicine:**

AI analyzes patients' genomic data to identify genetic markers that may influence treatment response Ashley (2016); Collins & Varmus (2015). This is particularly useful in oncology, where genetic variations can impact how patients respond to specific treatments Hood & Friend (2011).

Example: For cancer patients, AI can analyze the genetic makeup of a tumor to determine the most effective chemotherapy agents, reducing unnecessary side effects and increasing treatment efficacy.

4. **Optimizing Medication Dosage and Timing:**

AI-based systems personalize medication dosages based on individual patient metrics, including body weight, age, metabolic rate, and drug interactions Rajkomar et al. (2019). AI can also suggest optimal medication schedules to enhance efficacy and reduce side effects Miotto et al. (2018).

Example: In hypertension management, an AI system can analyze blood pressure trends and adjust medication timing or dosage to achieve target blood pressure levels while minimizing side effects .

5. **Lifestyle Recommendations and Behavioral Interventions:**

AI-driven recommendations often include lifestyle changes, such as diet adjustments, exercise plans, and stress management techniques Ashley (2016). It can watch for adherence and adjust these recommendations based on real time data Rajkomar et al. (2019).

Example: An AI-driven platform may advise patients with Type 2 diabetes of a daily step goal, and track physical activity through wearables. Activity patterns used by the AI allow goals to be adjusted or motivational props to be given.

4.3 Examples of AI Improving Treatment Accuracy and Patient Outcomes

1. Diabetes Management:

Case Study: Diabetic patients can use this AI powered mobile app integrated with AI to track their glucose levels, track dietary habits and adjust insulin dosages.

The app, which offers real time insights and feedback, ensures that patients stay in stable glucose levels that prevent complications such neuropathy and retinopathy.

Impact: Using AI supported treatment plans, patients experience better glucose control and fewer hypoglycemic episodes, while increasing overall quality of life.

2. Cancer Therapy Personalization:

Case Study: In oncology AI algorithms use tumor genomics to recommend the most targeted therapies to each patient based on their genetic profile. As an example, an AI powered platform can help oncologists select from different chemotherapy regimens that match the molecular structure of a tumor, which can improve the chances of a treatment working.

Impact: Personalized treatment is associated with higher remission rate, less side effects and better survival outcome than generalized treatment strategies.

3. Heart Disease Management:

Case Study: Likewise, continuously tracking heart rate and blood pressure movements is a task for AI powered wearable devices. Analyzing this data, AI can help recommend personal tolls on medications, lifestyle changes, or even warn patients to check with a physician if they experience symptoms of arrhythmia or other heart problems.

Impact: Heart conditions patients are far less likely to visit the emergency room and monitor their long term health better as their treatment is adjusted based on real time data.

Figure 8. Personalized Treatment Planning Workflow with AI

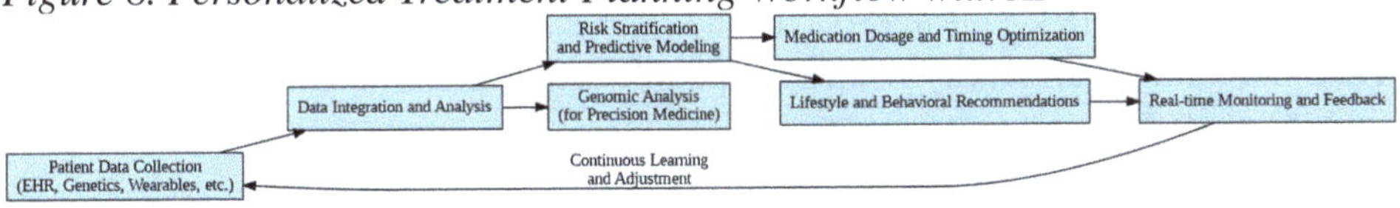

4.4 Benefits of Personalized Treatment Planning with AI

1. **Improved Treatment Accuracy:**

Treatment adjustments driven by AI ensure that they're precise to each patient's unique biology and will increase the likelihood of success Topol (2019); Rajkomar et al. (2019).

2. **Enhanced Patient Outcomes:**

After all, personal treatments are formulated to minimize side effects, reduce complications, and ultimately achieve better long term health outcomes for patients Ashley (2016); Collins & Varmus (2015).

3. **Increased Patient Engagement:**

Personalized recommendations help make patients more engaged in their care because it shows the relevance and impact on your treatment for you, personally Bodenheimer & Sinsky (2014).

4. **Reduction in Healthcare Costs:**

By identifying which interventions to implement, and which to avoid, AI avoids unnecessary treatments that lead to hospitalizations, costing less to patients and healthcare providers Miotto et al. (2018); Rajkomar et al. (2019).

With AI delivered personalized treatment planning, chronic disease management moves from reactive to proactive, to personalized for each patient's specific characteristics Topol (2019). This approach is a major leap forward in obtaining optimal health outcomes and quality of life for people with chronic conditions Morley et al. (2020).

5 ENHANCED DIAGNOSTICS WITH AI

5.1 Early Detection Diagnostic Algorithms

Artificial Intelligence (AI) is changing diagnostics through highly accurate, fast and timely disease detection Topol (2019); Rajkomar et al. (2019). Early diagnosis is equally important for chronic disease like diabetic retinopathy and cancer, where early treatment instills average opportunity to improve work results as well as to decrease risk associated with harsh complications Esteva et al. (2017); Miotto et al. (2018). Machine learning and deep learning are used in AI driven diagnostic algorithms to analyze the complex medical data to help provide evidence that allows clinicians to detect conditions at a time when it is very early in its onset with a system that could detect the condition even before the symptoms show Rajkomar et al. (2019); Topol (2019). In this section we look at AI based diagnostic algorithms and their use in the field of chronic disease detection including how AI can be used to favor provision of accurate and premature diagnosis Miotto et al. (2018).

Early Detection Diagnostic Algorithms, medical images x-ray, MRI, CT scan, or retinal scans have been very popular for deep learning learning with a high matching precision Esteva et al. (2017). Diabetic retinopathy and cancer, where early intervention can significantly improve patient outcomes and reduce the risk of severe complications Topol (2019); Rajkomar et al. (2019). AI-driven diagnostic algorithms use machine learning and deep learning to analyze complex medical data, helping clinicians detect conditions at their earliest stages, often before symptoms appear Miotto et al. (2018). This section explores AI-based diagnostic algorithms, their application in chronic disease detection, and the benefits of AI for achieving accurate and early diagnosis Topol (2019).

5.2 Diagnostic Algorithms for Early Detection

1. **Image-Based Diagnostics with Deep Learning:**

Deep learning models, particularly Convolutional Neural Networks (CNNs), have proven to be highly effective in analyzing medical images, such as X-rays, MRIs, CT scans, and retinal images Esteva et al. (2017); Miotto et al. (2018).

Example: In diabetic retinopathy detection, CNNs analyze retinal fundus images to identify micro aneurysms, hemorrhages, and other abnormalities associated with early stages of retinopathy. This allows for prompt intervention to prevent vision loss .

Example: In oncology, deep learning models analyze mammograms and CT scans to detect small lesions or abnormalities that may be indicative of early-stage cancer, providing the basis for early treatment.

2. **Natural Language Processing (NLP) for Analyzing Clinical Text:**

NLP algorithms extract relevant information from clinical notes, radiology reports, and pathology records, enabling healthcare providers to identify disease patterns that may otherwise go unnoticed Rajkomar et al. (2019); Miotto et al. (2018).

Example: NLP models analyze electronic health records (EHRs) to flag high-risk patients based on prior symptoms, medical history, and lab results . For example, patients with family history indicators of cancer or cardiovascular disease may be flagged for further screening .

3.**Biomarker Analysis Using Machine Learning:**

Machine learning models analyze biomarkers (molecules found in blood, tissues, or fluids) to detect the presence of disease or the risk of future complications Ashley (2016); Hood & Friend (2011).

Example: In cancer diagnostics, AI-based models evaluate genetic mutations, proteins, and other biomarkers to predict cancer risk and help in early diagnosis. This is especially beneficial in conditions like breast and lung cancer, where biomarkers are critical indicators of disease

4.**Predictive Analytics in Diagnostics:**

Predictive analytics models assess patient data to estimate the likelihood of developing certain conditions based on risk factors such as age, lifestyle, and genetic history Rajkomar et al. (2019); Miotto et al. (2018).

Example: AI models analyze patient data to predict the likelihood of developing Type 2 diabetes based on factors such as BMI, family history, and lifestyle. Patients identified as high-risk can be guided toward preventive measures to delay or prevent disease onset.

5. **Wearable Devices and Remote Monitoring for Diagnostics:**

AI algorithms process data from wearable devices, like heart rate monitors, glucose sensors, and ECGs, for continuous health monitoring and early detection of abnormalities Keesara et al. (2020); Miotto et al. (2018).

Example: Wearables paired with AI driven ECG analysis can detect arrhythmias, heart rate variability, and other irregularities in patients with cardiovascular disease, alerting the patient and healthcare provider early on in the disease process .

5.3 Benefits of AI in Accurate, Early Diagnosis

Artificial Intelligence in Medical Diagnostics: Precision and Accessibility

1. **Enhanced Diagnostic Accuracy**

AI systems are designed to process vast amounts of medical data with incredible precision Topol (2019); Rajkomar et al. (2019). By minimizing human error stemming from fatigue, bias, or oversight, AI contributes to more reliable diagnostic outcomes Miotto et al. (2018). This is especially important in fields that rely on image interpretation, such as radiology and pathology Esteva et al. (2017).

Example: AI tools have been shown to detect breast cancer from mammograms with accuracy comparable to, or better than, trained radiologists. This technology supports medical professionals by adding an extra layer of accuracy in diagnosing complex conditions .

2. **The Role of AI in Early Detection**

Early detection is critical for improving treatment success rates Collins & Varmus (2015). When chronic diseases are identified in their initial stages, less invasive treatments can often be employed, preventing disease progression Ashley (2016).

Example: AI systems used to analyze retinal scans can identify early indicators of diabetic retinopathy .Early diagnosis enables timely treatment, such as laser therapy or medication, which can help prevent vision loss .

3. **Accelerated Diagnostic Processes**

AI's ability to analyze medical data at high speeds facilitates rapid diagnostics, which is crucial in busy healthcare settings or in areas with limited specialist availability Miotto et al. (2018); Keesara et al. (2020).

Example: AI-powered diagnostic tools can review chest X-rays in seconds, identifying early signs of conditions like pneumonia . This allows clinicians to begin treatment promptly, reducing complications and improving outcomes .

4. **Cost Efficiency in Healthcare**

Diagnosing diseases early with AI reduces the need for advanced, invasive treatments, which are often more expensive Bodenheimer & Sinsky (2014). This not only saves healthcare costs but also alleviates the financial burden on patients Miotto et al. (2018).

Example: Early cancer detection through AI may result in less aggressive treatments, thereby lowering overall treatment expenses and hospitalization costs .

5. **Improved Accessibility in Remote Areas**

AI is playing a significant role in expanding access to healthcare Bashshur et al. (2014). With the help of telemedicine platforms and portable AI-enabled devices, quality diagnostics can reach rural and underserved areas Keesara et al. (2020).

Example: AI-driven portable ultrasound machines can be operated by non-specialists in remote regions, with AI software interpreting the scans to provide actionable insights. This addresses gaps in healthcare access where trained professionals are scarce .

6. **Continuous Learning for Better Outcomes**

AI models are not static; they evolve by integrating new data, allowing them to refine their diagnostic capabilities over time Rajkomar et al. (2019). Regular updates from clinical studies and patient records ensure that AI tools remain accurate and effective Miotto et al. (2018).

Example: In oncology, updated datasets help AI systems identify patterns in imaging and pathology, resulting in improved accuracy for detecting progressive stages of cancer .

Figure 9. AI-Enhanced Diagnostic Workflow

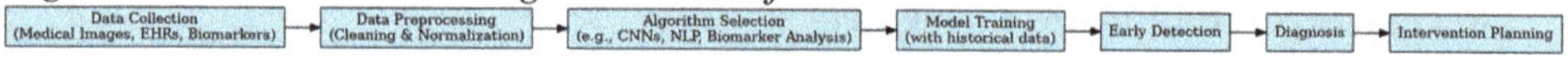

5.4 Case Studies Highlighting AI in Diagnostics

- **Diabetic Retinopathy:**

AI tools analyzing retinal images help identify early signs of the disease Rajkomar et al. (2019); Esteva et al. (2017). These systems are particularly valuable in resource-limited settings, where specialists may not be available Bashshur et al. (2014).

Outcome: Early intervention reduces the likelihood of vision loss in diabetic patients Topol (2019).

- **Oncology:**

AI enhances cancer detection by analyzing mammograms and biopsy slides for abnormalities Esteva et al. (2017); Ashley (2016).

Outcome: Early-stage cancer diagnosis improves survival rates and reduces the need for aggressive treatments Hood & Friend (2011); Collins & Varmus (2015).

- **Cardiac Health Monitoring:**

Wearable devices embedded with AI technology can track heart rate and detect irregularities signaling potential cardiovascular issues Topol (2019); Keesara et al. (2020).

Outcome: Alerts generated by these devices encourage timely medical intervention, preventing severe events like strokes or heart attacks Bodenheimer & Sinsky (2014).

Artificial intelligence is reshaping modern healthcare by delivering accurate, accessible, and efficient diagnostic tools Topol (2019); Rajkomar et al. (2019). Its ability to detect diseases early, reduce costs, and expand care to underserved areas makes it a vital asset in both preventive medicine and chronic disease management Miotto et al. (2018); Bashshur et al. (2014).

6. AI IN MEDICATION MANAGEMENT FOR CHRONIC DISEASES

An AI driven medication management system is reshaping chronic disease care by improving medication adherence, maximizing dosage and real time monitoring Rajkomar et al. (2019); Topol (2019). Predictive analytics, machine learning, and data integration from different sources (e.g., electronic health records, patient reported outcomes, wearable devices) are used these systems to furnish a more precise and based on feedback medication management procedure Miotto et al. (2018). This proactive model is necessary for the guidance of chronic disease including diabetes, hypertension, cardiovascular disease, among others, where consistent medication adherence and tailored dosing will have a huge impact on patient outcome Collins & Varmus (2015); Ashley (2016).

Limitations and Challenges of AI in Chronic Disease Management:

AI holds significant promise for transforming chronic disease management; however, it encounters various limitations Morley et al. (2020). Key among these are the necessity for extensive, high-quality datasets, which are not always readily accessible Miotto et al. (2018); the potential for algorithmic bias that may reinforce existing disparities in healthcare Mittelstadt et al. (2016); and concerns surrounding data privacy and patient consent Morley et al. (2020). It is essential to tackle these challenges to guarantee the fair and effective implementation of AI in the healthcare sector Topol (2019).

6.1 Medication Management Systems Using Automated Systems

Automated medication management systems use AI to support various functions:

1. Medication Adherence Tracking:

AI systems track how patients adhere to prescribed regimens, notice patterns of missed doses and electronically send reminders through apps or text message Bodenheimer & Sinsky (2014); Rajkomar et al. (2019). Suppose some example of this is an intelligent digital pill organizer with an AI algorithm telling the patient when to take their medications and informing the caregivers if meds have been skipped Miotto et al. (2018).

2. Predictive Analytics for Dosage Adjustments:

Health data trends can inform AI when a patient will require a dosage change Topol (2019). One example is for diabetes management, as AI can, for example, look at blood glucose readings coming in from wearable sensors and suggest how much insulin to adjust accordingly Rajkomar et al. (2019).

3. Adverse Drug Interaction Monitoring:

A patient's full medication profile can be leveraged to identify potential drug interactions that an AI algorithm can use to help avoid adverse effects Ashley (2016). AI uses multiple sources such as a patient's medical history, medication records and known interaction databases to improve patient safety Collins & Varmus (2015).

4. Inventory and Refill Management:

The medications can be monitored by automated systems to see when there's not enough and alert patients or caregivers to get prescriptions refilled before they're run out Bashshur et al. (2014). Other systems tie right into pharmacies, making the process automatic and keeping essential medications readily available Keesara et al. (2020).

6.2 AI Applications in Monitoring and Optimizing Medication Regimens

1. **Personalized Dosage Recommendations:**

Taking all of those data and sucking it through the AI to try to find those dosage recommendations that are tailored for an individual is where this kind of research is at Rajkomar et al. (2019); Miotto et al. (2018). In hypertension, for instance, AI can adjust dosages depending on real-time blood pressure readings and aims to respond instantaneously to it by reducing side effects Topol (2019).

2. **Continuous Monitoring and Adjustment:**

AI integration with wearable devices will monitor physiological parameter constantly and then take adjustments to medication on the spot Keesara et al. (2020). Take attention, e.g. in asthma management, AI powered inhalers with sensors could help track usage patterns, understand the external effect and suggest ways to prevent an asthma attack Rajkomar et al. (2019).

3. **Data-Driven Medication Regimen Optimization:**

By using patient data to design the best possible drug or drug combination to treat a disease the system eliminates the need for multiple medications while maximizing the chance of delivering a maximal positive drug outcome Ashley (2016); Hood & Friend (2011). It is particularly useful in patients with multiple chronic disease that may require polypharmacy (administration of multiple drugs) Collins & Varmus (2015).

4. **Predictive Alerts for Non-Adherence:**

It has the power to recognize behavioral patterns and identity barriers that may interrupt adherence allowing for proactive intervention Bodenheimer & Sinsky (2014). For instance, if a system recognizes in a week's time that a patient has missed more than a few doses, it can notify a healthcare provider so he or she can check up on the patient and determine, if any, what may be holding the dose back: side effects, access issues etc. Rajkomar et al. (2019).

Table 3. AI-Driven Medication Management Applications

AI Application	Description	Example
Medication Adherence Tracking	Monitors adherence patterns, sends reminders, and notifies caregivers of missed doses	Digital pill organizers alerting patients to take medications
Predictive Dosage Adjustments	Uses health data to adjust dosages in real-time	Insulin adjustments based on blood glucose data from continuous monitoring devices
Adverse Drug Interaction Alerts	Identifies potential drug interactions based on patient profiles	AI algorithms analyzing patient history and current medications
Inventory & Refill Management	Tracks medication supply and automates prescription refills	Automated reminders for refills linked with pharmacy systems
Personalized Dosage Recommendations	Customizes dosage based on EHR, genetic data, and real-time health metrics	Blood pressure medication adjustments based on real-time blood pressure readings
Continuous Monitoring	Analyzes wearable data to optimize medication timing and dosage	AI-driven inhalers tracking usage and advising on asthma management
Predictive Alerts for Non-Adherence	Uses behavioral data to predict non-adherence, enabling timely provider intervention	Alerts to healthcare providers when patients miss multiple doses

Figure 10. AI-Driven Medication Management Workflow

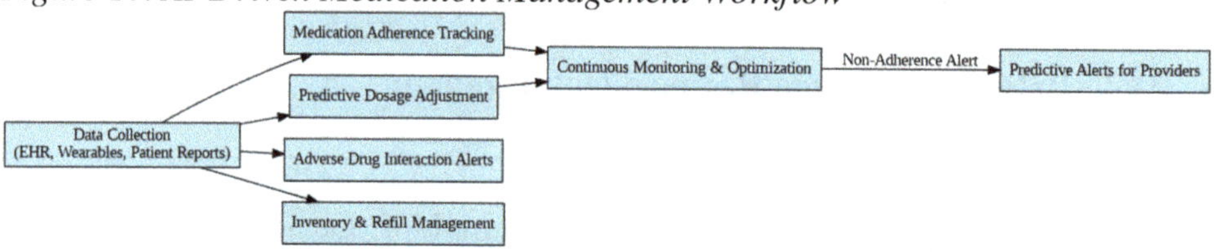

7. TELEMEDICINE AND REMOTE MONITORING WITH AI

Telemedicine and remote monitoring have become a transformative field for AI in which healthcare providers are able to more effectively manage chronic disease outside of traditional clinical settings Topol (2019); Bashshur et al. (2014). For patients living with chronic conditions, requiring long term management, continued monitoring, real time data analysis and personalized interventions becomes possible, with AI supporting telemedicine Rajkomar et al. (2019); Miotto et al. (2018). AI powered wearables help patients get monitored remotely at home, decreasing the visits at the hospital and helping with the accessibility and convenience of healthcare Keesara et al. (2020).

7.1 How AI Enhances Telehealth and Remote Patient Management

1. Automated Data Collection and Analysis:

The information (Vital signs and other health metrics) is collected by AI driven telemedicine platforms from wearables and mobile devices so a healthcare provider can continuously monitor them Miotto et al. (2018); Rajkomar et al. (2019). With this data being processed in real time, AI algorithms can find patterns and sniff out anomalies which could suggest a complication, and early identification of these issues can often be correlated with a better outcome Topol (2019).

Example: Wearable device that tracks blood pressure and heart rate is being monitored by AI to monitor cardiovascular health .The system can alert the patient, warns healthcare providers if an abnormal heart rate is detected.

2. Personalized Alerts and Notifications:

Each patient's baseline health metrics are analyzed by AI systems to define set personalized thresholds Rajkomar et al. (2019). Systems send alerts to the patient and the care team if any metric, other than the baselines, deviates more than significantly Miotto et al. (2018). It allows for quick intervention which minimises the risk of the complication Topol (2019).

Example: The AI system notifies a diabetic patient wearing a continuous glucose monitor (CGM) when blood sugar levels spike or go dangerously low, and then take immediate action to balance out the blood sugar.

3. Predictive Analysis for Preventive Care:

Historical data is fed to the o AI models to predict if a person might develop some health issue in the future Rajkomar et al. (2019); Miotto et al. (2018). This predictive capability can be used to prevent early intervention in preventing the occurrence of chronic diseases, and reducing emergency hospitalizations Topol (2019).

Example: Unlike traditional systems that often require extensive training or supervision, an AI system can help a chronic obstructive pulmonary disease (COPD) patient have their respiratory patterns analyzed and able to predict an impending exacerbation such that early interventions, like medication adjustment or lifestyle changes, can be initiated.

4. Teleconsultations with AI-Enhanced Insights:

In virtual consultations, AI helps healthcare providers find their way through it, analyzing patient data and suggesting possible diagnosis or treatment in real time Rajkomar et al. (2019). It speeds up the consultation process and makes sure providers are sitting with all the information that they need Topol (2019).

Example: By analyzing recent health data of a patient's wearable device, AI processes this data and presents the doctor with an overview during a virtual consultation in order to make an accurate and efficient diagnosis and treatment adjustments .

5. Behavioral and Lifestyle Support:

Operated by AI driven telehealth platforms, behavioral and lifestyle advice is provided based on an AI driven data view Ashley (2016). This includes alerts for medication, exercise parameters and additional dietary implications of the 'minor medical farm' Bodenheimer & Sinsky (2014).

Example: As real-time blood pressure monitoring and activity tracking become available for a hypertensive patient, AI might suggest a low sodium diet or let the patient know to take a short walk if they've been sedentary .

6. Reduced Strain on Healthcare Facilities:

At the same time AI powered telemedicine enables remote management of chronic diseases allowing that much fewer visits and admissions to hospital especially for routine check ups and follow up, freeing more resource for more serious cases Bashshur et al. (2014); Keesara et al. (2020).

Example: Wearable devices in use daily for monitoring and feedback provide patients with heart failure fewer frequent in person checks unless a critical issue arises due to infection .

7.2 The Role of AI in Wearables for Real-Time Data Collection and Patient Tracking

1. **AI-Enabled Wearable Devices for Continuous Health Monitoring**

They include tracking of vital signs that include heart rate, blood pressure, respiratory rate and oxygen levels, continuously, using the power of AI Topol (2019); Keesara et al. (2020). tory rate, and oxygen levels continuously. The metrics on these are processed in real time so that healthcare providers can have a continuous information on a patient's health status Miotto et al. (2018).

Example: Wearable ECG monitors sense arrhythmias and signal potential problems early Topol (2019). Active wearables such as accelerometers and gyroscopes on wearables can monitor patient activity levels, steps and even detect falls Bashshur et al. (2014). piratory rate, and oxygen levels continuously. These metrics are processed in real-time, allowing healthcare providers to gain a continuous view of the patient's health status Rajkomar et al. (2019).

Example: Wearable ECG monitors detect arrhythmias and provide early warnings of potential heart conditions.

2. **Activity Tracking and Mobility Monitoring:**

Wearables equipped with accelerometers and gyroscopes can monitor patient activity levels, steps, and even detect falls Keesara et al. (2020). Basing mobility on activity data and tracking exercise routines: as a result, AI analyzes activity information to evaluate mobility and then health care providers are alerted if there is an unexpected drop in activity levels Miotto et al. (2018).

Example: An elderly patient's mobility can rapidly decline and AI can notify a care team so there can be further investigation into possible health issues.

3. **Sleep Quality and Stress Monitoring:**

In managing conditions like cardiovascular disease and diabetes, o AI algorithms analyze sleep patterns, duration and quality Ashley (2016). Of course AI can also sense stress based on heart rate variability and other biomarkers Topol (2019).

Example: For diabetics, the device is a wearable that tracks a patient's sleep stages and the AI provides feedback on how sleep quality impacts blood glucose levels, making suggestions for lifestyle changes .

4. **Medication Adherence and Management:**

Some wearables (such as devices) and their AI powered mobile apps remind patients to take a medication and track there adherence Rajkomar et al. (2019). AI monitors medication schedules to help keep people on track with the medication that is needed to manage a chronic disease effectively Miotto et al. (2018).

Example: For a hypertensive patient, an AI driven app sends a reminder to take medication and sends follow up notifications if a dose was missed .

5. **Integration with EHR for Comprehensive Care:**

With AI integrated wearables, data can automatically be synced to Electronic Health Records (EHRs) and clinicians can get the big picture of a patient's health and make more informed decisions Rajkomar et al. (2019); Miotto et al. (2018).

Example: Data from wearables is collected continuously and brought into the patient's EHR so doctors can see trends and adjust treatment plans .

Figure 11. AI-Enhanced Telemedicine and Remote Monitoring Workflow

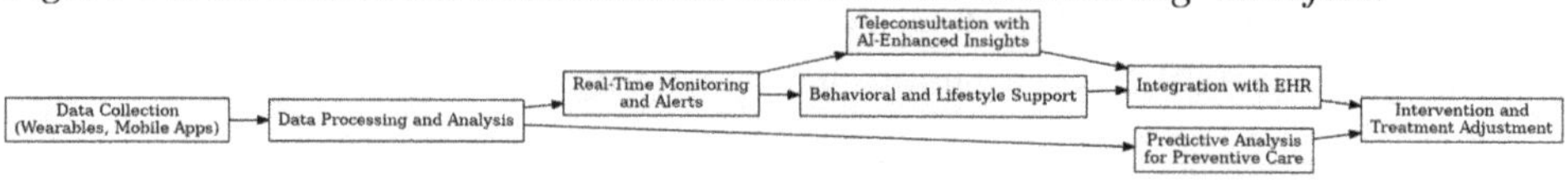

Table 4. AI Applications in Telemedicine and Remote Monitoring

AI Application	Description	Example
Vital Sign Monitoring	Tracks heart rate, BP, respiratory rate, oxygen levels	Continuous ECG monitoring for arrhythmia
Activity and Mobility Tracking	Monitors physical activity and detects falls	Alerts for sudden drops in mobility
Sleep Quality and Stress Detection	Analyzes sleep patterns and stress indicators	Feedback on sleep quality affecting glucose
Medication Adherence	Reminds patients to take medication and tracks compliance	Notifications for missed doses
Predictive Health Alerts	Predicts complications based on historical and real-time data	Early COPD exacerbation alert
Teleconsultation Support	Provides data insights for virtual consultations	Summary of recent health metrics for doctors
EHR Integration	Syncs wearable data with EHR for comprehensive patient records	Trend analysis in EHR for decision-making

7.3 Benefits of AI-Enhanced Telemedicine and Remote Monitoring

1. Timely Interventions:

All potential health issues are caught and brought up immediately for real time alerts through continuous monitoring Topol (2019); Rajkomar et al. (2019).

2. Improved Patient Engagement:

Patients are given personalized reminders, alerts, and feedback, all of which help keep patients in the driver's seat when it comes to their own care Bodenheimer & Sinsky (2014); Ashley (2016).

3. Enhanced Access to Care:

Telemedicine powered by AI is a great way to make healthcare accessible for patients in remote or underserved areas, so you don't have to travel to the doctor's office Bashshur et al. (2014); Keesara et al. (2020).

4. Reduction in Hospital Readmissions:

This remote monitoring means that problem is too early detected then you used to have unnecessary hospital admissions and the reduction in health care cost Topol (2019); Miotto et al. (2018).

5. Data-Driven Decision Making:

Having a picture of the patient's health from real time data from wearables integrated to EHR allows healthcare providers form more informed and precise treatment plan Rajkomar et al. (2019); Miotto et al. (2018).

Telemedicine and remote monitoring with AI at the core enables healthcare providers to provide proactive, personalized and efficient care, and forms the cornerstone of modern chronic disease management Topol (2019). In addition to improving patient outcomes, these systems also offer a sustainable approach to healthcare by optimizing resources and extending care beyond the clinical setting Bodenheimer & Sinsky (2014); Morley et al. (2020).

7.3 Benefits of AI-Enhanced Telemedicine and Remote Monitoring

1. Timely Interventions:

All potential health issues are caught and brought up immediately for real time alerts through continuous monitoring Topol (2019); Rajkomar et al. (2019).

2. Improved Patient Engagement:

Patients are given personalized reminders, alerts, and feedback, all of which help keep patients in the driver's seat when it comes to their own care Bodenheimer & Sinsky (2014); Ashley (2016).

3. Enhanced Access to Care:

Telemedicine powered by AI is a great way to make healthcare accessible for patients in remote or underserved areas, so you don't have to travel to the doctor's office Bashshur et al. (2014); Keesara et al. (2020).

4. Reduction in Hospital Readmissions:

This remote monitoring means that problem is too early detected then you used to have unnecessary hospital admissions and the reduction in health care cost Topol (2019); Miotto et al. (2018).

5. Data-Driven Decision Making:

Having a picture of the patient's health from real time data from wearables integrated to EHR allows healthcare providers form more informed and precise treatment plan Rajkomar et al. (2019); Miotto et al. (2018).

Telemedicine and remote monitoring with AI at the core enables healthcare providers to provide proactive, personalized and efficient care, and forms the cornerstone of modern chronic disease management Topol (2019). In addition to improving patient outcomes, these systems also offer a sustainable approach to healthcare by optimizing resources and extending care beyond the clinical setting Bodenheimer & Sinsky (2014); Morley et al. (2020).

8 BENEFITS OF REAL-TIME DATA COLLECTION FOR CHRONIC DISEASE MANAGEMENT

1. **Early Identification and Prevention**

Continuous monitoring facilitates the early identification of potential health concerns prior to their escalation, enabling timely action from both patients and healthcare providers Topol (2019); Rajkomar et al. (2019). This approach is essential in managing chronic diseases to prevent complications that may necessitate emergency interventions Miotto et al. (2018).

For instance, real-time monitoring of heart rate and rhythm can identify arrhythmias in patients with heart disease, allowing for immediate treatment and reducing the likelihood of hospitalization Keesara et al. (2020).

Additionally, wearable devices can serve as reminders for medication compliance or treatment frequency, helping patients adhere to their prescribed regimens Bodenheimer & Sinsky (2014).

For example, in the case of heart disease patients, continuous monitoring of heart rhythm can detect arrhythmias and prompt timely intervention, thereby minimizing the risk of serious complications Topol (2019).

2. **Enhanced Medication Compliance**

AI-powered wearable devices serve as reminders for patients to take their medications and track adherence trends Rajkomar et al. (2019). This feature is especially advantageous for managing chronic illnesses such as hypertension or diabetes, which necessitate rigorous medication regimens Ashley (2016); Collins & Varmus (2015).

For instance, these wearables notify users when it is time to take their medication and log adherence, thereby promoting consistency in their treatment protocols Miotto et al. (2018).

3. **Personalized Care Through Data Utilization**

The utilization of real-time data gathered from wearable devices empowers healthcare professionals to dynamically customize treatment plans, aligning interventions with the specific health trends of each patient Topol (2019); Rajkomar et al. (2019).

For instance, continuous glucose monitoring (CGM) provides individuals with diabetes the ability to modify their dietary choices, insulin administration, and physical activity in real-time, thereby enhancing blood sugar regulation and minimizing the risk of complications Collins & Varmus (2015); Ashley (2016).

Additionally, AI-enhanced wearables, such as gait analysis tools, evaluate movement patterns over time, allowing for further customization of treatment according to individual requirements Miotto et al. (2018).

For example, real-time glucose monitoring removes uncertainty in diabetes management, facilitating accurate modifications to insulin and activity levels based on immediate data Topol (2019).

4. **Improved Patient Involvement and Empowerment**

Wearable devices enable patients to gain immediate access to their health data, encouraging them to actively engage in the management of their health conditions Bodenheimer & Sinsky (2014).

For instance, individuals with hypertension can utilize real-time blood pressure measurements to make timely modifications, such as decreasing salt consumption or enhancing physical activity Ashley (2016).

Such involvement allows patients to make well-informed choices concerning their lifestyle and treatment options, ultimately leading to better health outcomes Collins & Varmus (2015).

5. **Decreased Healthcare Expenses**

AI-powered wearable devices enhance the early detection of health concerns and support remote monitoring, thereby minimizing the need for hospital visits and emergency treatments Bashshur et al. (2014); Keesara et al. (2020).

For instance, wearables that monitor respiratory rate and SpO_2 levels can identify early exacerbations in patients with COPD, allowing for outpatient management rather than expensive emergency care Rajkomar et al. (2019).

Furthermore, ongoing monitoring offers a comprehensive perspective on health metrics, which assists in timely interventions and lowers overall healthcare costs Miotto et al. (2018).

For example, COPD patients utilizing wearables for SpO_2 tracking can prevent recurrent hospitalizations by proactively managing exacerbations Topol (2019).

6. **Enhanced Management of Chronic Diseases via Trend Analysis**

Ongoing monitoring yields valuable insights into long-term patterns, allowing healthcare professionals to make informed modifications to treatment protocols Rajkomar et al. (2019); Miotto et al. (2018).

For instance, wearable devices that track heart rate variability over extended periods assist healthcare providers in fine-tuning medication, dietary choices, or exercise regimens to improve the management of heart disease Topol (2019).

By utilizing trend analysis, healthcare providers can anticipate possible complications and enhance treatment approaches based on both historical and real-time data.

Figure 12. Real-Time Monitoring Workflow with AI-Enabled Wearables

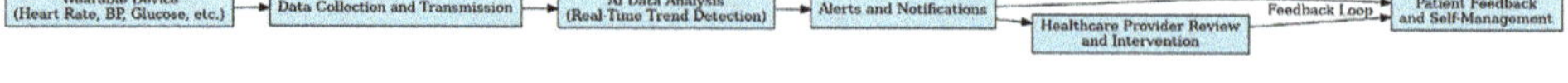

Table 5. Common AI-Enabled Wearables and Their Health Metrics

Wearable Device	Health Metrics Monitored	AI-Enabled Features	Common Uses in Chronic Disease Management
Apple Watch	Heart rate, ECG	Arrhythmia detection, personalized activity	Cardiovascular disease, stress management
Omron HeartGuide	Blood pressure, heart rate	Blood pressure trend analysis, hypertension alerts	Hypertension management
Dexcom G6 CGM	Glucose levels	Predictive glucose alerts, trend analysis	Diabetes management
Fitbit Sense	Heart rate, SpO2, respiratory rate	Sleep quality analysis, stress monitoring	COPD, sleep apnea, general wellness
Oura Ring	Heart rate variability, sleep stages	Readiness scores, stress level analysis	Cardiovascular health, sleep quality improvement
WHOOP	Physical strain, recovery, HRV	Personalized activity recommendations	Exercise and recovery monitoring for heart disease

9. ETHICAL AND PRIVACY CONSIDERATIONS IN AI FOR HEALTHCARE

Growing up, AI will increasingly become part of healthcare, and ethical and privacy considerations need to be addressed Topol (2019); Morley et al. (2020). To reap the benefits but without disadvantaging any user groups, AI is supported in the realm of healthcare settings to ensure that data is private, that AI algorithms are not biased for one group; and that the healthcare resource is equally accessible by everyone Mittelstadt et al. (2016); Morley et al. (2020). These issues must be addressed in order to protect vulnerable populations, maintain patient trust and improve care quality Bodenheimer & Sinsky (2014).

9.1 Issues Related to Data Privacy and Security in AI Applications

1. Sensitivity of Healthcare Data

Challenge: Healthcare data encompasses Protected Health Information (PHI), including medical histories, diagnoses, and genetic information, all of which are extremely sensitive Mittelstadt et al. (2016). Breaches of confidentiality can result in discrimination, stigmatization, and a deterioration of trust in healthcare systems Morley et al. (2020).

Example: A data breach that reveals patients' HIV status or mental health records may lead to discrimination in employment opportunities or insurance coverage .

2. Data Ownership and Control

Challenge: Patients frequently find themselves without control over the utilization of their health data once it has been collected by healthcare providers or AI platforms Morley et al. (2020). Ethical dilemmas arise when AI systems collect data for algorithm development without adequately informing patients about the potential future applications of that data Mittelstadt et al. (2016).

Example: The absence of informed consent regarding data collection and its subsequent use can undermine patient autonomy and erode trust .

3. Cybersecurity Risks

Challenge: AI systems that depend on cloud storage are susceptible to hacking, which can result in significant data breaches Topol (2019).

Example: A cyberattack targeting an AI-based diagnostic platform could jeopardize patient records, diminishing trust and revealing sensitive information .

4. Data Anonymization Challenges

Challenge: Anonymized data remains at risk of re-identification, particularly when dealing with extensive datasets that contain distinctive attributes Morley et al. (2020).

Example: Even datasets that have been anonymized can facilitate the identification of uncommon medical conditions or specific demographic groups, thereby threatening patient privacy .

5. Need for Consent and Transparency

Requirement: Patients should have the right to grant or revoke consent regarding the use of their data Morley et al. (2020).

AI systems must provide clear information about the analysis and utilization of data Topol (2019).

Example: Patients may decline to share their data if they are not informed about its intended use, underscoring the necessity for transparent consent processes .

Table 6. Ethical and Privacy Considerations and Proposed Solutions

Consideration	Description	Proposed Solution
Data Privacy and Security	Protecting sensitive health information from unauthorized access	Implement robust encryption and access control measures
Data Ownership and Control	Ensuring patients have control over their health data	Allow patients to opt-in and withdraw data sharing
Algorithm Bias	Avoiding skewed model outputs that harm specific populations	Use diverse datasets and fairness algorithms
Equitable Access	Ensuring AI tools are accessible to all patient demographics	Deploy low-cost wearables and telemedicine solutions
Algorithm Explainability	Providing clear, interpretable model decisions	Develop explainable AI to enhance provider understanding
Informed Patient Consent	Educating patients on AI's role in care	Ensure clear communication and consent processes

10. ETHICAL AND PRIVACY-CONSCIOUS AI IN HEALTHCARE

1. **Ensure Transparent Data Usage**:
   - o Clearly inform patients about the scope of data collection, storage, and analysis, and allow them to make informed choices about participation.
2. **Use Fairness Techniques in AI Models**:
   - o Apply fairness and bias detection algorithms during model training to ensure balanced representation across different demographic groups.
3. **Protect Data Security with Advanced Encryption**:
   - o Implement advanced encryption and secure access protocols to safeguard data from unauthorized access and potential breaches.
4. **Enable Explainability for AI Models in Healthcare**:
   - o Use interpretable AI techniques to ensure healthcare providers understand AI's decision-making process, allowing for accountability and verification.
5. **Improve Accessibility and Affordability**:
   - o Ensure AI-driven healthcare tools, such as wearables, are affordable and accessible, particularly in underserved and low-income communities.
6. **Conduct Regular Audits and Assessments**:
   - o Regularly evaluate AI systems for biases, security vulnerabilities, and performance across diverse patient groups to maintain fairness and reliability.

Ethical and privacy considerations are central to the responsible deployment of AI in healthcare. By prioritizing patient data security, addressing algorithmic bias, and fostering transparency, healthcare providers and AI developers can work toward creating equitable, trustworthy, and effective AI-driven healthcare solutions.

Figure 13. Future Outlook for AI in Chronic Disease Management

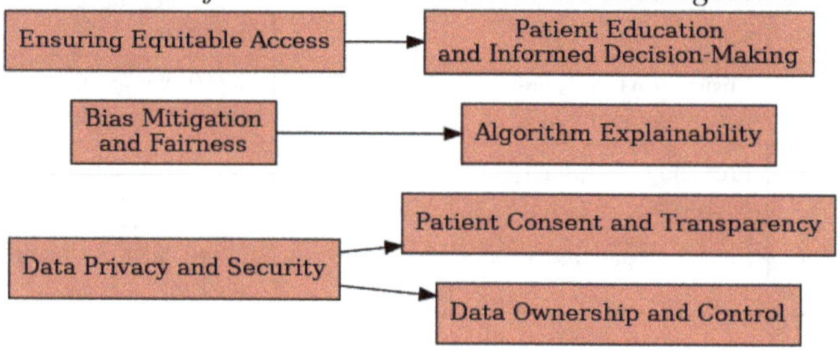

Now, chronic disease management will become much more efficient with all hands on deck including AI. Rising healthcare system reliance on AI for early detection, personalised treatment, remote monitoring and data drive decision making bodes well for the future of improving chronic disease management outcomes. Transformative changes in how chronic diseases are diagnosed, managed, and prevented are coming thanks to advancements in AI technology and collaboration between healthcare providers, technology innovators and policymakers.

11. THE ROLE OF AI IN SHAPING THE FUTURE OF HEALTHCARE SYSTEMS

1. Preventive and Predictive Healthcare:

The future of healthcare will transition from reactive treatment to a focus on preventive care and AI will increasingly guide the shift in focus for healthcare Topol (2019); Rajkomar et al. (2019). Predictive models will leverage real time data from wearable and patient records to predict potential health issues before becoming obvious, for preventive intervention Miotto et al. (2018).

Example: Continuous health data will be analyzed by the AI algorithms to predict the risk of a patient developing heart failure or worsening kidney disease and provide early preventive measures prior to emergency hospitalizations Topol (2019).

2. Personalized Medicine:

As a result, AI will be used to bring personalized treatment plan based on a patient's genetic, lifestyle and medical data to minimize the treatment effect. With the help of AI, precision medicine will provide tailored interventions to meet the needs of people with chronic disease .

Example: AI systems will be able in diabetes care to recommend specific diets, exercise plans, and doses of medication based on real time glucose monitoring, lifestyle factors and the patient's unique response to treatment .

IBM Watson Health utilizes artificial intelligence to assess patient information and suggest cancer therapies by examining genetic characteristics, lifestyle elements, and medical backgrounds, thereby enhancing treatment results while reducing adverse effects .

3. Enhanced Remote Monitoring and Telemedicine:

As AI enabled wearables and telemedicine advance, remote monitoring will be at the core of chronic disease management Keesara et al. (2020); Bashshur et al. (2014). It will enable patients to manage their conditions from home while continuing to get high quality care, advantageous for those in rural or underserved populations Bashshur et al. (2014).

Example: AI powered wearables will monitor chronic respiratory diseases in real time using lung function, oxygen levels and environmental factors, and alert patients and healthcare providers if there is evidence of an exacerbation.

4. AI-Driven Decision Support Systems for Healthcare Providers:

By providing clinical decision support to healthcare providers, AI will increase the accuracy and confidence of data driven decisions with which they make Rajkomar et al. (2019). At the patient level, AI will use analysis of patient data to diagnose, recommend treatment options, predict outcome, and so forth Miotto et al. (2018).

Example: In oncology, AI will enable the oncologists by analysing the tumor characteristics and genetic profile to recommend personalized therapies with the highest probability of success on similar cases.

5. Improved Resource Allocation in Healthcare:

In healthcare, AI will assist in allocating resources more efficiently through a capability of identifying high risk patients that need intensive monitoring and intervention and ultimately, improving care efficiency and lowering costs Bodenheimer & Sinsky (2014); Rajkomar et al. (2019).

Example: They can also use predictive algorithms to compute which patients are likely to end up in the hospital to enable the use of capacity effectively, and to therefore allocate resources to those who have the most pressing needs.

6. **Seamless Data Integration Across Healthcare Systems:**

Essentially, AI will enable patient data interoperability across many different healthcare platforms, so that providers have a holistic view of a patients' health history, real time metrics, and results of treatment Miotto et al. (2018); Rajkomar et al. (2019). The integrated approach will help make collaboration between different specialists easier, and patient care simpler Topol (2019).

Example: AI enabled EHR would automatically sync data from wearables, lab results and patient reported outcomes for providing a unified health record accessible to all care providers involved in care of a patient.

12. COLLABORATION AMONG HEALTHCARE PROVIDERS, TECHNOLOGY INNOVATORS, AND POLICYMAKERS

1. **Developing Ethical Standards and Guidelines**:

Ethical standards for AI use in healthcare will be established by policymakers who will also ensure that AI applications are patient privacy, data security, and ethical guidelines are respected.. The collaboration will contribute to the existing public trust in AI and help to promote broader adoption of AI in healthcare.

Example: In the long term, we believe that governments and healthcare organizations can help form a regulatory framework for how AI should behave ethically, such as bias mitigation, patient consent and data security standards.

2. **Innovating with Multidisciplinary Partnerships**:

To implement effective AI in health, we must work together; health providers, data scientists, engineers, and medical researchers together must develop the AI tools that are clinically viable and patient centered..

Example: The AI firms can work with hospitals to jointly create diagnostic algorithms for chronic diseases that utilize the feedback from clinician for improving usability and clinical accuracy.

3. **Investment in AI Training and Education for Healthcare Workers**:

This implies that health care providers will require training in the use and interpretation of AI generated insights so that maximum benefits of AI for chronic disease management can be achieved.. Targeted educational programs can support this and policymakers and technology innovators can.

Example: Training programs for hospitals in using AI tools for diagnostics and support will be provided, so healthcare professionals know what AI can and cannot do in clinical practice.

4. **Expanding Access to AI-Driven Healthcare in Rural and Underserved Areas**:

There are ways policymakers can incentivize and subsidize the use of AI driven healthcare specifically that of rural and underserved areas.. By ensuring that the benefits of AI in chronic disease management reach more people, we have achieved distribution.

Example: Such funding could be channels by governments towards telemedicine in rural areas to help those with chronic diseases access AI based remote monitoring and consultation from home.

5. **Promoting Interoperability Between AI Systems and Healthcare Platforms**:

In order for AI to be successful, there must be interoperability between AI tools, EHRs, and other systems of healthcare.. This means technology innovators, healthcare providers and policymakers collaborating to create standards that fly when it comes to sharing data.

Example: The best design of such an AI enabled platform will include integration with the patient's primary health care provider's EHR to allow the provider to have real time access to all of the patient data.

6. **Encouraging Research and Development in AI for Healthcare**:

In order to foster AI innovation in healthcare, healthcare researchers should be funded and incentives should be given for companies that develop AI solutions supporting chronic disease management.. Support for this can speed breakthroughs and grow AI's reach.

Example: Grants on from governments may be provided on companies researching AI solutions to early disease detection and prevention of chronic diseases which can electrify innovation and factor overall the healthcare ecosystem.

Table 7. Key Areas in the Future Outlook of AI for Chronic Disease Management

Area of Focus	Description	Expected Benefits
Preventive and Predictive Care	AI shifts focus to prevention by predicting disease risks	Reduced complications and improved patient outcomes
Personalized Medicine	Customizes treatments to individual health profiles	Optimized treatments and minimized adverse effects
Remote Monitoring	Uses wearables and telemedicine for continuous patient care	Lower hospital visits and enhanced patient convenience
Decision Support	Provides insights for healthcare providers	Informed, data-driven decision-making in chronic disease care
Resource Allocation	Prioritizes high-risk patients for interventions	Efficient use of healthcare resources
Data Integration	Integrates data from various sources into one system	Comprehensive patient care and improved data accuracy
Ethical Standards	Establishes regulations to ensure responsible AI use	Increased public trust in AI for healthcare
Multidisciplinary Partnerships	Collaboration across fields for AI development	Clinically relevant, patient-centered AI tools
AI Training and Education	Trains healthcare workers to use AI tools	Effective adoption of AI in clinical settings
Expanded Access	Makes AI-driven healthcare accessible in underserved areas	Equitable healthcare and improved outcomes in all regions
Interoperability	Ensures compatibility between AI and healthcare systems	Streamlined data flow and comprehensive health records
Research Funding	Government incentives for healthcare AI research	Accelerated innovation and better chronic disease solutions

12.1 Area of Focus Description Expected Benefits

Preventive and Predictive Care: The application of AI facilitates a shift towards preventive measures by assessing disease risk, thereby reducing complications and enhancing patient outcomes.

Personalized Medicine: Treatments are tailored to individual health profiles, resulting in optimized therapies with minimal adverse effects. The integration of wearable and telemedicine enables remote patient monitoring, reducing the need for hospital visits and providing more convenient care.

Decision Support: AI offers valuable insights to healthcare providers, promoting informed and data-driven decision-making in the management of chronic diseases.

Resource Allocation: The system prioritizes high-risk patients for timely interventions, ensuring an efficient allocation of healthcare resources.

1. Data Integration: Consolidation of data from multiple sources into a unified system enhances patient care and improves data accuracy.
2. Ethical Standards: Establishing guidelines for the responsible use of AI fosters increased public trust in AI applications within healthcare.

AI Development: Collaboration across various disciplines leads to the creation of clinically relevant, patient-centered AI tools.

AI Training and Education: Healthcare professionals are trained to effectively utilize AI tools, facilitating the adoption of AI in clinical environments.

AI-driven healthcare initiatives aim to reach underserved populations, ensuring equitable access to healthcare and improved outcomes. The interoperability of AI systems ensures compatibility with existing healthcare infrastructures, streamlining data flow and maintaining comprehensive health records.

During the government retreat, my session focused on identifying potential research funding opportunities to promote healthcare AI research, which will accelerate innovation and enhance solutions for chronic diseases.

12.2 Key Recommendations for a Collaborative Future in AI for Chronic Disease Management

1. **Foster Interdisciplinary Collaboration**:

Clinically useful, patient-centered, and ethically sound, AI tools should be created by healthcare provider, technologist, and policymaker collaboration.

2. **Standardize Ethical and Regulatory Frameworks**:

This will augment wat the public trust in AI and responsible use in healthcare by creating awareness of ethical guidelines that will prioritize patient privacy, data security and transparency..

3. **Encourage Accessible AI Solutions**:

Promote AI infrastructure that reaches underserved populations by providing AI wearable and telemedicine platform through government funding and incentives..

4. **Promote Interoperability Standards**:

This would enable o the development of interoperable systems, so that AI tools seamlessly interoperate with electronic health records and other healthcare system, such that data can flow smoothly.

13. INVEST IN AI RESEARCH AND EDUCATION

Education of healthcare providers on AI tools will have a role to play in ensuring that the tools ar effectiveness taken in patient care and funding of AI research will promote innovation..

AI in chronic disease management has a bright future in a healthcare environment that is based on data driven, personal and preventive. AI has the ability to change healthcare quality, accessibility and outcomes of the patients with chronic diseases worldwide, with the help of the collaborative work between healthcare providers, technology innovators and policymakers.

REFERENCES

Ashley, E. A. (2016). Towards precision medicine. *Nature Reviews. Genetics, 17*(9), 507–522. PMID: 27528417

Bashshur, R. L., Shannon, G. W., & Smith, B. R.. (2014). The empirical foundations of telemedicine interventions in primary care. *Telemedicine Journal and e-Health, 20*(5), 342–375. PMID: 27128779

Bodenheimer, T., & Sinsky, C. (2014). From triple to quadruple aim: Care of the patient requires care of the provider. *Annals of Family Medicine, 12*(6), 573–576. PMID: 25384822

Collins, F. S., & Varmus, H. (2015). A new initiative on precision medicine. *The New England Journal of Medicine, 372*(9), 793–795. PMID: 25635347

Esteva, A., Kuprel, B., & Novoa, R. A.. (2017). Dermatologist-level classification of skin cancer with deep neural networks. *Nature, 542*(7639), 115–118. PMID: 28117445

Hood, L., & Friend, S. H. (2011). Predictive, personalized, preventive, participatory (P4) cancer medicine. *Nature Reviews. Clinical Oncology, 8*(3), 184–187. PMID: 21364692

Keesara, S., Jonas, A., & Schulman, K. (2020). Covid-19 and health care's digital revolution. *The New England Journal of Medicine, 382*(23), e82. PMID: 32240581

Miotto, R., Wang, F., Wang, S., Jiang, X., & Dudley, J. T. (2018). Deep learning for healthcare: Review, opportunities, and challenges. *Briefings in Bioinformatics, 19*(6), 1236–1246. PMID: 28481991

Mittelstadt, B. D., Allo, P., Taddeo, M., Wachter, S., & Floridi, L. (2016). The ethics of algorithms: Mapping the debate. *Big Data & Society, 3*(2), 2053951716679679.

Morley, J., Machado, C. C., Burr, C., Cowls, J., Joshi, I., Taddeo, M., & Floridi, L. (2020). The ethics of AI in health care: A mapping review. *Social Science & Medicine, 260,* 113172. PMID: 32702587

Rajkomar, A., Dean, J., & Kohane, I. (2019). Machine learning in medicine. *The New England Journal of Medicine, 380*(14), 1347–1358. PMID: 30943338

Topol, E. J. (2019). High-performance medicine: The convergence of human and artificial intelligence. *Nature Medicine, 25*(1), 44–56. PMID: 30617339

Chapter 6

Systematic Review of Medical Imaging and Clinical Data in CKD Prediction Using Deep Neural Networks

Dattatray G. Takale
https://orcid.org/0000-0002-8241-3989
Vishwakarma Institute of Technology, India

Mahesh Shinde
Avantika University, Ujjain, India

Parikshit N. Mahalle
https://orcid.org/0000-0001-5474-6826
Vishwakarma Institute of Technology, India

Surendra Rahamatkar
https://orcid.org/0000-0002-1211-0560
Avantika University, Ujjain, India

Gopal Deshmukh
https://orcid.org/0009-0009-9975-8877
Vishwakarma Institute of Technology, India

ABSTRACT

The global healthcare problem of chronic kidney disease (CKD) requires accurate predictions in the early stages to achieve appropriate treatment and management

DOI: 10.4018/979-8-3373-0179-2.ch006

t © 2026, IGI Global Scientific Publishing. Copying or distributing in print or electronic forms without written permission of IGI Global Scientific Publishing is prohibited. Use of this chapter to enerative artificial intelligence (AI) technologies is expressly prohibited. The publisher reserves all rights to license its use for generative AI training and machine learning model development.

strategies. Deep learning through deep neural networks (DNNs) has received rising interest for CKD prediction systems because it effectively combines medical images with clinical information. The review investigates the implementation of deep neural networks for predicting CKD by uniting medical imaging approaches with clinical database information. Medical imaging techniques using ultrasound as well as CT scans and MRI, together with clinical datasets, generate important information regarding the initial development stages of CKD. The enormous computing ability of DNNs makes them perfect for detecting intricate patterns that standard evaluation techniques typically overlook. The article investigates multiple DNN structures predicting CKD, system performance levels, obstacles, and possible future enhancements.

1. INTRODUCTION

The main characteristic of CKD as a global health concern is progressive deterioration or complete loss of kidney function over time (Islam et al., 2023). The condition includes structural defects, persistent urine abnormalities, and excretory renal dysfunction from lost functional nephrons (Debal & Sitote, 2022). The sustained decline of glomerular filtration rate below 60 mL/min/1.73 m2 for three months or more suggests both impairment and improper functioning of the kidneys (George et al., 2022). The worldwide distribution of CKD extends from every corner of the earth. Yet, low- and middle-income countries bear maximum disease intensity, and they have minimal capacity to fight this condition. According to reports, 800 million people experience this ailment in every part of the world (Pal, 2023). The prevalence rate of CKD has increased by 29.3% for all age groups throughout three decades. The age-standardized DALYs rate steadily rose at a rate of 0.30 EAPC up to 514.86/100,000 by 2019, alongside an increasing age-standardized incidence rate reaching 233.65/100,000 through a 0.69 EAPC by 2019 (Sawhney et al., 2023). The World Health Organization (WHO) has forecasted that CKD will become one of the five most widespread persistent conditions in 2040. The condition now ranks among the primary sources of mortality because it has caused increased death tolls during the previous two decades (Antony et al., 2021).

The progression of CKD results in end-stage renal disease, which medical professionals consider an individual risk factor for heart disease and accelerated mortality patterns (Ramspek et al., 2021). Glomerulonephritis, along with diabetes mellitus type 1 and hypertension, make significant contributions to worldwide increases in CKD development (Khalid et al., 2023). The functional decline of kidneys observed in older adults constitutes a considerable risk factor because aging involves cellular changes such as telomere attrition, genomic instability, autophagy, inflammation, modifications to Sirtuin and Klotho signaling pathways, and mitochondrial function

(Praveen et al., 2024). The research indicates these elements are key controllers affecting kidney aging progress. The combination of obesity's production of oxidative stress with inflammation, adverse hemodynamic effects, and renin-angiotensin-aldosterone system activation makes obesity a critical risk factor that advances CKD (Rashed-Al-Mahfuz et al., 2021).

The relationship between non-alcoholic fatty liver disease and CKD has been reported in numerous populations recently (Akter et al., 2021). Since early disease manifestations usually remain undiscovered, they extend treatment delays, thus contributing to increased mortality statistics (Almustafa, 2021). Early diagnosis is the best way to prevent CKD advancement and its related complications. The healthcare system has experienced a revolution because of artificial intelligence (AI), especially in its ability to discover early kidney-related diseases (Bai et al., 2022).

Modern medical applications of artificial intelligence through machine learning and deep learning methods now serve as both strong and practical tools that enable newer possibilities of risk assessment, early diagnosis, and tailored treatment plans to enhance patient results (Ferguson et al., 2022). The massive dataset of genetic data combined with EHRs and essential clinical information helps AI algorithms detect hidden relationships that human analysts usually cannot see (Sitaraman et al., 2024). AI serves multiple research functions by improving patient results and enabling rapid medical actions while forecasting the initial development stages of renal disease. The developed models provide exact outcomes to reduce kidney disease burden effectively. Early healthcare professionals can leverage AI tools to integrate analytical innovations into practice, allowing for a more effective diagnosis and prevention of kidney disease onset in the early stages (Kumari & Singh, 2022). The developed predictive models demonstrate the potential to enhance disease diagnosis and provide medical practitioners with better options for quality patient care. Disease categorization and prediction utilize two algorithms: random forests and artificial neural networks, which are the most common in practice (Iftikhar et al., 2023). Machine learning algorithms use medical photo analysis to identify the best treatment options based on clinical patient populations, which leads to enhanced kidney disease diagnosis capabilities. Physicians gain real-time patient health monitoring through remote systems, whereas predictive analytics helps doctors detect patients who face health threats (Geng et al., 2024).

This study emerged from the critical requirement to improve preventive CKD patient care and more innovative therapy strategies. The interface capabilities of artificial intelligence help clinical decision-making provide better real-time insights about complicated data, which leads to better patient outcomes. The future of CKD prognosis research will advance because AI models can direct new studies that develop this field. The review study examined the existing research thoroughly while presenting a prognosis summary of CKD and describing the latest developments and neglected aspects for upcoming investigations. Research findings will demonstrate how essential artificial intelligence systems are for changing CKD management, making them a key factor in improving patient quality of life.

2. MATERIALS AND METHODS

The systematic review implemented the PRISMA principles to ensure proper reporting quality. The research utilized PubMed, ScienceDirect, The Cochrane Library, Google Scholar, and Scopus databases while prioritizing content published within 2024. The study used Boolean operators to locate relevant documents relating to CKD combined with terms describing deep learning, machine learning, and artificial intelligence. Clinical settings utilized AI-based prediction models (deep learning or machine learning) to detect and predict the advancement of CKD. The researchers executed model comparisons, leading to result assessments that included accuracy, specificity, and sensitivity reporting. The PICO framework was used to select the studies through evaluation methods, which included patients with CKD (P), AI-based prediction models (I), comparison with other models (C), and pertinent outcome metrics (O). The analysis limited itself to peer-reviewed English studies regarding interventions and clinical trials, randomized controlled trials (RCTs), non-RCTs, and comparative studies. The research included only studies addressing acute renal illnesses while utilizing AI models with sufficient data and excluding case reports, letters, comments, abstracts from meetings, editorials, conference papers, protocols, reviews, or animal studies.

Figure 1. PRISMA analysis

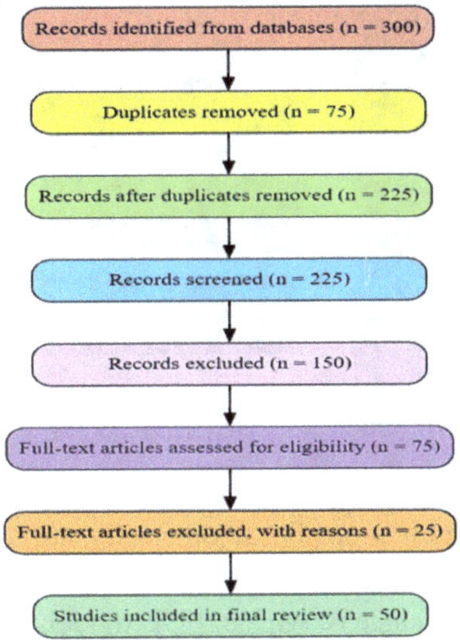

The article analyses CKD prediction tools by evaluating three major classification groups that combine optimization-based approaches with deep learning and machine learning methods. The present global patient count of CKD represents a progressive and irreversible condition, yet early detection enables better medical outcomes and decreased healthcare costs. Researchers have developed systems with early-stage CKD prediction capabilities because data-driven methods allow them to utilize clinical demographic and laboratory data. The increased use of machine learning techniques occurred through their accessible interfaces, interpretable approaches, and affordable implementation of SVM, Decision Trees, Random Forest, and k-nearest Neighbours (k-NN). Multiple complex medical patterns in extensive data sets can be identified better by deep learning models, which include LSTM networks and CNN and RNN architectures.

Figure 2. Plan of review

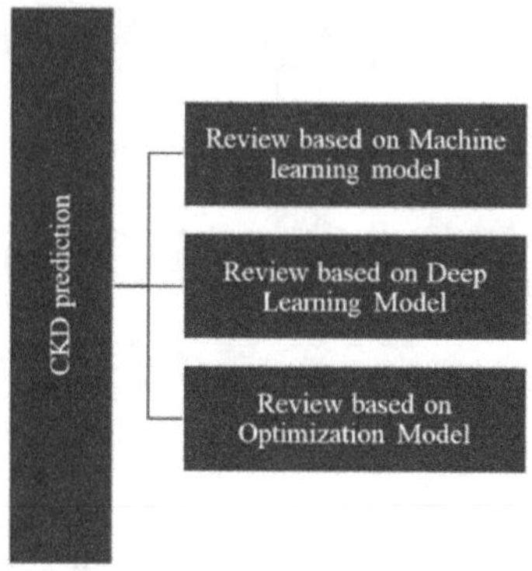

The number of implementations based on optimization methods such as hybrid optimization frameworks, metaheuristics, and evolutionary algorithms continues to rise to enhance the performance of ML and DL models (Mehta et al., 2024). The predictive models' predictive power and generalization level increase when these techniques optimize hyperparameters and select features while optimizing model parameters. Researchers measure the anticipated model precision and computing speed, information processing capacity, resistance against failure, and practical value for clinical use within each category. This paper discusses challenges related to unbalanced data distributions, feature selection, and AI explainability needs in healthcare tasks (Jabbar & Rithanya, 2021). The research attempts to fully understand different categories using comparative analysis and this series of three groups. The study points out modern market trends that indicate the increasing need for mixed models that unite ML frameworks, DL approaches, and optimization methods to achieve better performance outcomes. This assessment presents future studies, clinical potential, and optimal strategies for predicting CKD in its concluding segment.

2.1. Review Based on Machine Learning Model

The section analyzes machine learning methods that identify CKD by assessing predictive models. Medical research entities demonstrate substantial interest in machine learning techniques because these methods analyze clinical data to conduct autonomous early diagnosis without human intervention. The models use CKD kidney disease patient training data to detect critical illness patterns linked with disease progression factors. Many studies have established that machine learning achieves outstanding prediction results through proper preprocessing, correct feature selection and validation, and required preprocessing methods. The models are valuable because they offer adjustable implementations across different healthcare data collections. The primary concerns in medical decision-making stem from data-related problems such as missing values, data imbalance, and the need for explanation. According to studies, adding domain expertise with refined data management practices is a research priority for experts because it enhances model reliability. Machine learning leadership in CKD prognosis improves healthcare assessment and specialized care plans.

The hybrid model mentioned by Navita et al. (Mittal et al., 2025) consists of four different stages. The Synthetic Minority Oversampling Technique-Edited Nearest Neighbors Rule is a combination sampling approach that applies data balancing solutions during the first model stage. The second stage combines five renowned datasets (Long Beach, VA, Hungarian and Switzerland and Statlog (Heart)) to select essential features through Chi-square analysis from 1190 clinical entries with 11 features. The system directs preprocessed data to a stacking ensemble model which implements Logistic Regression (LR) as a meta-learner with Grid Search Cross-Validation (GSCV) optimization methods and three base learners consisting of Random Forest Tree (RFT) and K-Nearest Neighbor (K-NN) and AdaBoost classifier. The ensemble model performance compares with the results achieved by its subcomponents.

An efficient method for CHD identification from ECG signals was shown by Adyasha Rath et al. (Rath et al., 2021) through their straightforward but reliable application of LSTM networks. The model analyzes ECG signal recordings of 268 participants present in the PTB diagnostic database version 1.0.0 PhysioNet. The developed detection model incorporates three stages of the LSTM network structure, where each stage contains 256, 128, and 64 modules while maintaining 20% weight random dropouts between modules. Two different training approaches for validation have been applied in both 70 and 30% proportions and 80 and 20% proportions.

A risk factor method used for coronary heart disease prediction was developed by Vardhan Shorewala et al. (Shorewala, 2021). The evaluation of predictive algorithms K-Nearest Neighbors and Binary Logistic Classification and Naive Bayes depends on accuracy and recall measurements with ROC curve analysis. Cluster modeling techniques consisting of bagging, boosting, and stacking methods evaluate the operations of individual classifiers. The study focused on understanding which ensemble methods improve the prediction accuracy rates for coronary heart disease diagnosis. Research using the "Cardiovascular Disease Dataset" based on patient records for coronary heart disease includes 70,000 subjects for evaluation. The average accuracy boost from bagged models reaches 1.96% more than standard models.

Identifying cardiac illness through machine learning methods receives detailed attention from E. Chandralekha et al.'s study (Chandralekha et al., 2023). The framework contains three significant elements: ensemble classifier training, data preprocessing, and feature selection. Experimental findings offer example-based proof of predictions by identifying key factors in the different classification models. Oldpeak and thali and ca, along with cp and that, define the significant features of Random Forest, while Gradient Boosting identifies ca and cp as well as that and old peak and age as key characteristics. The essential features shared among the models include data presented by AdaBoost and Extra Trees Classifier. Multiple verification techniques show that the Extra Trees Classifier delivers the highest accuracy among the models. The research implements valuable inspection algorithms to detect heart issues that should assist medical professionals during diagnosis decisions.

The proposed framework by Deepali Yewale et al. (Yewale et al., 2023) provides an efficient cardiac disease prediction framework through ensemble techniques that combine data balancing along with outlier detection and removal approaches while doing without feature selection. The Cleveland dataset provides data for 303 cases and is the research foundation obtained from the UCI repository. The UCI repository marks fourteen of seventy-six variables in the open-source dataset as critical heart disease risk factors. Random oversampling serves as a solution to deal with uneven data distributions. An isolation forest method exposes multivariate data outliers because its approach has not been studied before. A prediction model that incorporates bagging and boosting alongside voting and stacking approaches is created after disrupting anomalies from the dataset.

Table 1. Problem formulation of the machine learning models

Author(s)	Techniques Used	Outcome / Focus	Drawbacks / Limitations
Mittal et al., 2025	Hybrid Sampling, Chi-square, Stacking (RFT, K-NN, AdaBoost), Logistic Regression	Developed a robust 4-stage hybrid model for heart disease prediction using ensemble learning	It may require high computational resources and be limited to structured clinical datasets.
Rath et al., 2021	LSTM Network (3 layers),	Accurate detection of CHD using ECG signals and deep learning architecture	It depends on the quality of ECG signals; it is less interpretable for clinical practice
Shorewala, 2021	K-NN, Naive Bayes, Logistic Regression, Bagging, Boosting, Stacking	Ensemble models are shown to improve CHD prediction over individual classifiers	Limited improvement margin (~1.96%); potential overfitting in ensemble approaches
Chandralekha et al., 2023	Random Forest, Gradient Boosting, AdaBoost, Extra Trees	Comprehensive framework highlighting feature importance across classifiers	The dataset is not specified; feature dependence varies across models
Yewale et al., 2023	Isolation Forest, Ensemble Techniques (Voting, Bagging, Boosting)	Effective prediction without manual feature selection; incorporated anomaly removal	It uses a smaller Cleveland dataset (303 records), potential underfitting risk

continued on following page

Table 1. Continued

Author(s)	Techniques Used	Outcome / Focus	Drawbacks / Limitations
Alalawi & Alsuwat, 2021	Deep Neural Network, Random Forest, Gradient Boosting	Automated CVD detection using ML and DL; RF achieved the best performance	No detailed dataset disclosure; performance gap between datasets
Terrada et al., 2020	Supervised ML Classifiers, 10-fold Cross Validation	Developed MDSS for atherosclerosis with strong average performance	Focused mainly on UCI datasets; real-time adaptability not tested
Baghdadi et al., 2023	CatBoost, Feature Selection, Ensemble Methods	Early-stage CVD detection with high F1 and accuracy through optimized ML	Lack of clarity on dataset size; real-world validation not discussed
Mandula & Vijaya Kumar, 2024	ALAN, Adaptive Boosted Decision Fusion (ET-ABDF)	High-performance cardiac disease model with strong AUC and F1 metrics	It may involve complex configuration; model explainability is not detailed
Subasi et al., 2017	Random Forest, Multiple ML Classifiers	CKD detection using standard UCI dataset; RF showed the best accuracy	Focused only on a static dataset; comparison limited to few classifiers

Cardiac disease analysis and detection have become possible through the AI algorithms and deep neural networks that Hana H. Alalawi et al. (Alalawi & Alsuwat, 2021) have developed. This study employs two datasets, Deep learning networks and various classification models under machine learning, to create automated cardiovascular illness diagnosis. Accuracy, combined with precision, recall, and f-score, determined the evaluation criteria for the different models. Random Forest demonstrated its best model performance in heart disease with 94% accuracy and gradient boosting achieved its peak performance in cardiovascular disease with all measured parameters at 73% accuracy, recall and F1-score, and precision at 74%.

Oumaima Terrada et al. (Terrada et al., 2020) built a supervised machine learning medical diagnosis support system (MDSS) to apply automatic learning to each patient's clinical information for forecasting atherosclerosis. The proposed MDSS for atherosclerosis requires three Machine Learning (ML) classifiers as its prediction method. This paper relies on two datasets from Sani Z-Alizadeh and the UCI repository (Cleveland and Hungarian). The performance measures were calculated using accuracy, recall, and precision values. The recommended system's performance was improved by calculating Matthews' correlation coefficient and F1-score. The suggested model was assessed using 10-fold cross-validation methods, which produced a best accuracy average of 94%. The proposed approach contributes toward healthcare development by simplifying extensive clinical diagnostics of atherosclerosis disorders.

In their research, Nadiah A. Baghdadi et al. (Baghdadi et al., 2023) demonstrate that machine learning techniques have massive potential to advance clinical cardiovascular disease treatment practices. These methods decrease healthcare costs because expensive and lengthy clinical investigations and laboratory tests become unnecessary as they enable evidence-based clinical guideline development alongside management algorithm creation. New machine learning algorithms should be developed because they need to be reliable and effective at automatic variable selection and early heart disease detection, which will enable early prediction of CVDs. The proposed Catboost model reaches an average accuracy level of 90.94% and generates a rough F1-score of 92.3% in its results. The model reached maximum classification results, showing superior accuracy and precision compared to multiple state-of-the-art systems today.

The Ensemble Technique with Adaptive Boosted Decision Fusion (ET-ABDF) was developed by Aruna Mandala et al. (Mandula & Vijaya Kumar, 2024) to enhance its accuracy level. Using the ALAN technique makes important properties more recognizable for predictive modeling applications. A score of 89.00%, along with 89.80% recall, 88.0% accuracy, and 89.81% precision, confirm the superior capability of the ET-ABDF model to detect heart disease. The excellent AUC value of 96.21% proves effective group discrimination capability. The assessment shows the introduced method achieves better results than other tested algorithms could produce.

Abdulhamit Subasi et al. (Subasi et al., 2017) state that machine learning (ML) techniques can identify CKD. Machine learning algorithms excel at finding abnormalities across different physiological information, which they successfully implement into multiple classification operations. This study uses various ML classifiers to test experimental results through actual UCI Machine Learning Repository data compared to recently published research findings. The research demonstrates that random forest (RF) delivers high accuracy rates when detecting CKD patients, and the outcomes are presented through statistical measures and descriptive analysis.

2.2. Review based on the Deep Learning Model

The section evaluates research implementations using deep learning models for CKD prediction. Deep learning represents an artificial intelligence subfield that transforms into a robust tool that detects hard-to-spot but nonlinear connections in medical data. Low human intervention during feature engineering remains a distinctive advantage of deep learning models that process high-dimensional or raw information. Medical professionals have utilized deep learning algorithms to identify CKD from many datasets, including structured electronic health records, unstructured medical documents, and time-based laboratory results. Deep learning frameworks deliver superior prediction assessment along with accuracy performance whenever large datasets become accessible, according to studies. Such predictive models can identify small changes and time-based patterns that suggest possible medical disease developments. Deep learning algorithms produce their best outcomes after spending large amounts of computer resources and annotated data. Medical staff need clear explanations on how to use new equipment in healthcare, which black-box mechanisms can obstruct. Recent research studies focus on improving model transparency because they tackle the existing constraints while implementing attention strategies. Deep learning technology maintains its substantial potential for enhancing CKD prediction, although it retains its ability to model complex clinical relationships while making data-driven clinical choices.

The authors K. Ramu et al. (Ramu et al., 2025) introduced a hybrid model that combines a support vector machine (SVM) with a convolutional neural network (CNN) for enhanced prediction accuracy of CKD. The model performance improved when SVM classified features extracted by CNN. The extensive clinical dataset contained ten medical indicators and received SMOTE processing. Applying the hybrid CNN model exceeded monolithic SVM or Random Forest implementations, which achieved respective accuracies of 94.8% and 94.6%, thus reaching 96.8% accuracy. The model achieved perfect recall for identifying CKD patients since its value was 1.00. Despite excessive computational demands, the system performs highly, highlighting the necessity for clinical performance-enhancing optimizations.

The researchers of Youngmin Bhak et al. (Bhak et al., 2025) developed three models, which included eGFR-MMDL (multimodal deep learning that merged retinal images with urine dipstick data), eGFR-UDLR (logistic regression applied to urine dipstick data), and eGFR-RIDL (retinal image deep learning for estimated glomerular filtration rate calculations). The 2009 CKD-EPI (Chronic Kidney Disease Epidemiology Collaboration) equation calculated the crucial chronic kidney disease biomarker eGFR<60 mL/min/1.73 m2 for predicting all models. This investigation relied on a multicenter database containing a development set (65,082) and an external verification set (58,284) from individuals within the age range of 20–79 years. Saliency maps displayed model attention through deep learning supported by wide residual networks. The results depended on numerical variables according to sensitivity analysis.

Jingying Ma et al. (Ma et al., 2025) presented a deep learning-based dynamic kidney failure prediction model (KFDeep) for CKD patients. Predictions occur in real-time by processing all clinical marker information accessible within real EHR data. The research relied on three datasets with hospital patients from Yinzhou China EHRs, with 2,752 patients used for training and 917 patients for validation in the development phase, while the external validation used data from 934 PFH cohort patients at the Peking University First Hospital. The KFDeep model outperforms other models with an AUROC of 0.946 (95\% % CI: 0.922-0.970) on the internal validation dataset and 0.805 (95\% % CI: 0.763-0.847) on the external validation dataset. The KFDeep model consistently performs in simulation dynamic conditions as the AUROC value steadily increases with time. The SHAP results alongside hidden layer trends confirm accepted medical knowledge, whereas the calibration and decision curve confirm the model's safety for real clinical use.

Table 2. Problem formulation of the deep learning models

Author(s)	Techniques Used	Outcome / Focus	Drawbacks / Limitations
Ramu et al., 2025	Hybrid CNN-SVM, SMOTE	Achieved 96.8% accuracy; perfect recall (1.00) for CKD cases	High computational load; needs further optimization for clinical use
Bhak et al., 2025	eGFR-RIDL, eGFR-UDLR, eGFR-MMDL; Wide ResNet; saliency maps	Multimodal deep learning using retinal and urine dipstick data; strong performance on large multicenter datasets	Complexity in combining modalities; interpretability challenges
Ma et al., 2025	KFDeep (deep learning); SHAP, EHR-based data	Dynamic CKD prediction using real-time EHRs; high AUROC (0.946 internal, 0.805 external)	External AUROC is lower than internal; it requires longitudinal data
Van Slobbe et al., 2025	Multimodal CNNs; MIMIC and eICU data; clinical notes + structured data	Predicts acute kidney injury (AKI); AUROC up to 0.90; strong transportability	Depending on data modality, performance varies with missing SCr/urine output
Lakshmi et al., 2025	DNN-RF hybrid, TSVD with Dingo optimization, KNN imputation	Automated disease prediction with 96.2% accuracy; early diagnosis aid	Dimensionality reduction may lead to information loss; dependency on optimization algorithm
Iqbal et al., 2025	Reciprocal Domain Adaptation Network (RDAN), MMA, DML, Pyramid Pooling	Achieved 96.94% accuracy, high precision (98.81%), and AUC (99.35%) using cross-domain learning	Complexity in training requires diverse datasets for generalization
Burra et al., 2025	cDCGAN + CNN	Tackles class imbalance in CKD datasets; improved performance via GAN-based data augmentation	GAN training is unstable; the quality of generated data may affect outcomes
Iliyas et al., 2025	Multiple DL models (RNN, CNN, LSTM, AE, GRU, RBM), genetic data	Predictive modeling of diabetic kidney disease (DKD); deep insights into biomarkers and genetic factors	Model generalizability across populations not addressed; complex biological interpretation
Akhtar et al., 2025	CNN with an attention mechanism	Diagnoses kidney abnormalities with 99.87% accuracy; strong image classification	High performance on limited image dataset; lack of clinical validation
Chang et al., 2025	Biosensor (SPE chip), ANN; UA concentration detection via cyclic voltammetry	Integrated biosensor + ANN for early CKD risk prediction based on uric acid levels	Focused on a specific biomarker (UA), general CKD risk prediction needs broader feature inclusion

R. van Slobbe et al. (Van Slobbe et al., 2025) developed three convolutional neural network-based models using data from the Medical Information Mart for Intensive Care (MIMIC) database. The models used clinical factors, free-text notes, and principles from the Elsevier H-Graph system. The predictions made by our models achieved high accuracy levels, with AUROC scores ranging from 0.73 to 0.90. Researchers evaluated these models twice and once, including urine output and Scr as prediction variables. The prediction performance of combination models using clinical factor instruments with clinical notes mirrored the results obtained from clinical variable-only models when Scr and urine output were considered predictive indicators. Predictive capabilities improved by uniting different modalities while eliminating SCr and urine output from the analysis. The eICU dataset enabled external evaluation of the models, which relied solely on clinical factors and achieved satisfactory results in the new population (AUROC 0.68-0.77).

Kanchi Lohitha Lakshmi et al. presented the DNN-RF model in their work (Lakshmi et al., 2025). KNN and min-max normalization techniques preprocess illness-related information before K-Nearest Neighbor-based missing value replacement. TSVD operates as the data dimension minimization method on preprocessed data. Dingo optimization determines the best TSVD component quantity through its optimization process. The disease prediction occurs through a hybrid classifier composed of DNN-RF. The experimental research demonstrates that this recommended approach delivers 96% precision and 95% specificity together with 96.2% accuracy. This computational system helps medical staff get faster diagnoses, leading to early treatment delivery and decreasing mortality statistics.

Saeed Iqbal and his team proposed a Reciprocal Domain Adaptation Network (RDAN) to solve problems during CKD diagnosis (Iqbal et al., 2025). The combination of various datasets through the RDAN neural network model serves as a solution for tackling complex CKD diagnosis challenges. RDAN contains two essential elements: Mutual Model Adaptation (MMA) and Domain Model Learning. The MMA unit retrieves valuable features from diverse data sources using global and local pyramid pooling strategies. The DML unit uses semi-supervised domain-independent features to enhance representation learning by combining the MMA system properties. The reciprocal regularizer in RDAN enhances feature representation strength and domain knowledge-sharing capabilities for specific identification of CKD cases. Using RDAN produced notability in accuracy (96.94%) and precision (98.81%) measurements along with recall (98.73%) and F1-Score (98.88%) and area under the curve (AUC—99.35%) when applied to real-world datasets.

The small and unbalanced datasets affect the performance of Convolutional Neural Networks (CNN) models presented by Lakshmi Ramani Burra et al. through their demonstration of kidney disorder diagnosis (Burra et al., 2025). Researchers have developed three methods to address this problem: cost modification, undersampling, and oversampling. The methods utilize local data instead of examining minority class distributions, which creates their primary operational constraint. The chapter introduces the conditional Deep Convolutional Generative Adversarial Network (cDCGAN), which offers a fresh solution for managing uneven distribution in Kidney Disease Diagnostics datasets. Through the cDCGAN operation, new minority examples emerge that mimic actual data sequences. A CNN model receives training for assessing the cDGCAN augmentation technique while comparing it against standard data augmentation methods. Testing accuracy receives significant enhancement when using the CNN model trained with data from the cDCGAN-based augmentation.

The genetic bases of diabetic kidney disease and deep learning predictive models are explained in detail in a work published by Iliyas Ibrahim Iliyas et al. (Iliyas et al., 2025). The analysis investigates the relationship between genetic and environmental influences in complex diseases, focusing on understanding monogenic syndromes to explain pathogenesis. The authors attempt to use diverse deep learning models such as autoencoder, long short-term memory, convolutional neural networks, limited Boltzmann machines, recurrent neural networks, and gated recurrent units to predict clinical outcomes related to diabetic kidney disease—the research analyzes model usages together with topological designs for assisting the detection of potential biomarkers. Many studies have shown that Deep Learning effectively detects DKD while identifying biomarkers that help understand potential risk elements. The research study presents barriers and future guidance regarding applying DL methods in medical work for diabetic patients with renal disease alongside solutions for those obstacles.

Muhammad Nadeem Akhtar et al. provided a Convolutional Neural Network (CNN) with an attention mechanism in their research (Akhtar et al., 2025). The model identifies kidney abnormalities among the signs of renal disease by recognizing tumors, stones, and cysts. The validation method employed k-fold cross-validation on a database containing about 4000 images distributed across 1000 images per class. The proposed CNN with concentration model achieves a remarkable 99.87% accuracy rate for different renal illness detection. This version maintains critical components by simplifying both verbalization and operational steps.

CKD risk evaluation and Urine Acid assessment through a deep learning-based Artificial Neural Network (ANN) system are combined with a biosensor for measuring UA presence in stones, according to Yaw-Jen Chang et al. (Chang et al., 2025). An SPE chip acts as the biosensor by undergoing oxygen plasma modification to its surface topology. The cyclic voltammetry performs concentration detection for UA. The experimental results show a direct connection between the anodic peak current and UA concentration range from 0.15 to 5 mM. The biosensor implements an effortless surface treatment solution that is inexpensive to implement. The ANN system received training using the CKD dataset and literary data with age and creatinine as primary inputs.

2.3. Review based on the Optimization Model

The section presents an analysis of research that employed optimization-based systems to forecast CKD outcomes. The primary purpose of optimization techniques includes selecting optimal features while changing parameters and improving convergence efficiency to enhance predictive model performance. The successful application of optimization techniques helps solve problems relating to overfitting and class imbalance and improves prediction accuracy in CKD. Model training setups are evaluated to maximize the output quality of prediction results through these optimization methods. Researchers study various mathematical and nature-inspired optimization approaches to achieve three specific studies: dataset generalization enhancement, precision optimization, and error rate minimization. Due to particular conditions, optimization enables shorter training times, used computing complexity, and superior model functioning. The advantages of optimization-based models do not eliminate their requirement for extensive tuning, their reactions to problem dimensionality, and initial starting conditions. According to modern research, developing dependable CKD prediction systems depends heavily on optimization since these methods prove essential for hybrid platforms that integrate multiple prediction paradigms.

The published work by L. Jerlin Rubini et al. (Jerlin Rubini & Perumal, 2020a) introduces FFOA and MKSVM as a practical classification approach. In the beginning, FFOA operates to identify the optimal subset features from existing available features. MKSVM uses the processed medical data features to perform classification evaluation. The researchers utilized MATLAB to develop a model based on the proposed classification approach for CKD patients. The dataset gets tested using four different datasets from UCI machine learning repositories: Cleveland, Hungarian, Kidney Chronic, and Switzerland. Multiple parameters, including accuracy, sensitivity, specificity, positive and negative predictive values, false favorable rates, false negative rates, and additional measures, evaluate the performance of the recommended CKD classification method.

The research paper by J. Sulthan Alikhan et al. (Alikhan et al., 2023) introduces a Self-Attention Convolutional Neural Network enhanced with a Season Optimization Algorithm for CKD Diagnosis through IoT and Cloud Computing in Smart Medical Big Data Health Care System (SACNN-SOA-CKD-IoT-CC). Wearable devices and sensors operate as IoT devices that gather information. A diagnostic model for CKD constitutes one of the key applications of the self-attention convolutional neural network (SACNN). The SACNN lacks details about optimization methods that dictate proper parameters for CKD classification. Codes implemented in SACNN use the season optimization method (SOA) as their optimization tool.

Table 2. Problem formulation of the deep learning models

Author(s)	Techniques Used	Outcome / Focus	Drawbacks / Limitations
Jerlin Rubini & Perumal, 2020a	FFOA for feature selection, Multi-Kernel SVM for classification	Accurate CKD classification using selected optimal features	Limited to MATLAB simulation; lacks deep learning comparison
Alikhan et al., 2023	SACNN with Season Optimization Algorithm (SOA); IoT + Cloud-based data collection	Smart medical CKD diagnosis in big data environments	No baseline optimization model before SOA; potential latency with cloud integration
Rubini & Perumal, 2020	Grey Wolf Optimization (GWO) for feature selection, Hybrid Kernel SVM for classification	Improved CKD prediction accuracy through feature selection	Heavy dependence on MATLAB environment; limited scalability
Jerlin Rubini & Perumal, 2022	Oppositional Firefly Optimization for feature selection, Deep Neural Network for classification	Enhanced convergence and classification accuracy in CKD detection	DNN model complexity not discussed; no external validation set
Aprilianto, 2020	CFS and Binary PSO for feature selection, SVM for classification	Accuracy improved from 63.75% to 95% with feature selection combination	Lacks analysis of model generalizability; small dataset scope
Pradeepa & Jeyakumar, 2024	LSNN for attribute selection, Hybrid Atom Crow Optimization in Improved Deep Belief Network (IDBN)	Early and accurate CKD prediction with 98% accuracy	Training time and model complexity not addressed
Sara & Kalaiselvi, 2019	Ant Colony Optimization for feature selection, Extreme Learning Machine (ELM) classifier	Fast, accurate CKD detection with minimized computation	ELM limitations with dynamic datasets; data preprocessing challenges
Ismail, 2023	Snake Optimization for feature selection, Five ML classifiers	Dimensionality reduction and accurate early detection of CKD	Snake algorithm novelty may lack extensive benchmarking
Jacquline & Sudha, 2024	K-Means Clustering + EBO for feature selection, Improved ANN classifier (IANN), WFCM clustering	High-precision CKD classification (up to 98.9%) with zero misclassification	Computational complexity due to the multi-stage processing pipeline
Pavan Kumar et al., 2025	Bacterial Foraging Optimization (BFO) for feature selection, SMOTE + IQR preprocessing, Ensemble modeling	Balanced and optimized CKD prediction by removing irrelevant features and handling class imbalance	Ensemble model interpretability was not discussed; there is potential overfitting.

According to Rubini et al. (Rubini & Perumal, 2020), the hybrid kernel support vector machine (HKSVM) represents a classification model designed to detect the presence of CKD. Distributed algorithms have gained extensive popularity during this time because they serve many different application domains. Advanced medical data evaluation methods require greater knowledge and skills for prediction and reorganization tasks. Our system offers one-of-a-kind feature selection capabilities that help detect and predict CKD effectively. Most of the data preprocessing steps will target the source input data. The preprocessed data undergoes best-characteristic selection by implementing the grey wolf optimization (GWO) algorithm. The proposed method applies a Hybrid Kernel Support Vector Machine (HKSVM) to determine the presence of CKD after data classification. The simulation runs under MATLAB.

CKD diagnosis benefits from a new classification model featuring optimal feature selection through Jerlin Rubini Lambert et al.'s (Jerlin Rubini & Perumal, 2022) metaheuristic algorithms. During the preprocessing stage, the data containing missing values received elimination treatment. A statistical technique, the Oppositional FireFly Optimization method, selects the best features from which the disease can be categorized or predicted more effectively. With oppositional-based learning principles implemented in the FireFly algorithm, the convergence rate experiences an enhancement. Researchers proposed using Deep Neural Networks for classification because they sought to detect CKD. A study of the dataset assessed the performance measures such as sensitivity, accuracy, and specificity of the proposed feature selection classifier.

The research group of Doni Aprilianto et al. (Aprilianto, 2020) presented Binary Particle Swarm Optimization (BPSO) for application. BPSO employs the highest fitness value for the selection of attributes. SVM accuracy enhancement as a result of merging CFS with BPSO constitutes the primary objective of this investigation. The prediction accuracy of SVM achieves 63.75% in the diagnosis of CKD. The 10 executed SVM algorithms with combined CFS and BPSO feature selection achieved an average accuracy rate of 95%, and SVM algorithms with just CFS feature selection obtained 88.75% accuracy. The diagnostic accuracy of CKD increases by 31.25% when using CFS and BPSO together as attribute selection methods for SVM.

The Local Search With Nearest Neighbor (LSNN) optimization method, which P. Pradeepa et al. (Pradeepa & Jeyakumar, 2024) developed, selects the most important attributes needed for deep net model training. The suggested LSNN optimization computes mean square error values through K-fold cross-validation while using them as fitness functions for local search optimization to discover optimal features. IDBN operates with chosen attributes resulting from the training process. The training system in IDBN uses atom crow optimization as a hybrid approach to enhance the traditional Deep Belief Network (DBN) performance. The assessment of several scenarios showed that the selected 15 attributes reached 98% accuracy and a 2% mistake rate through analysis. Combining LSNN-based attribution features with proposed deep learning produces optimal results for early-stage CKD prediction.

Research on CKD detection through S. Belina Ant Colony Optimization (ACO) Based Feature Selection and Extreme Learning Machine (ELM) was published by

V.J. Sara et al. (Sara & Kalaiselvi, 2019). Due to its characteristics, ELM has established a unique training system for immediate implementation in categorization divisions. Functionality optimization of ELM does not face many restrictions. The network can use the original ELM training procedure when identifying the ELM classifier space. The experiment proves the ELM classifier produces superior results than conventional methods like random input weight extraction. The study consists of 400 participants, among which 250 have CKD, and 150 do not, and the data contains missing and noisy entries. A new method to explore CKD leveraging the ELM technique with shorter computational time and accuracy suitable across different cost-accuracy trade-offs will be developed through future analysis.

The Snake-Efficient Feature Selection-Based Framework for Accurate Early Detection of CKD was created by Walaa N. Ismail et al. (Ismail, 2023). The feature selection method reduces dimensionality while enhancing model performance and overcoming the dimensionality curse. Blackbox optimization technology enabled natural-inspired optimization algorithms to become popular problem representation solutions through direct application for complicated situations. Researchers developed snake optimization algorithms that explore the hunting behavior of snakes to identify optimal or near-optimal solutions for complex problems. The primary purpose of this paper is to develop CKD-SO, which represents a revolutionary snake-optimized framework dedicated to CKD data analysis. Using five machine learning algorithms with snake optimization (SO) methods, researchers analyze and select the optimal medical data, leading to an accurate kidney and liver disease prediction.

M. Lincy Jacquline et al. (Jacquline & Sudha, 2024) developed a classification framework for CKD through EBO-IANN, which utilizes enhanced butterfly optimization and improved artificial neural network methods. Both preprocessing and feature selection processes utilize the K-means clustering (KMC) while Weighted Fuzzy C-means (WFCM) performs clustering and IANN handles classification. The authors conducted EBOIANN testing on the CKD dataset present at the UCI repository. Careful assessment demonstrates that the framework performs better than Bayesian algorithms and both Neural Networks (NN) and Modified K-means Support Vector Machine (MKSVM) and Enhanced Adaptive Neuro-Fuzzy Inference System (EANFIS). The EBO-IANN enhanced all assessment metrics, including accuracy, precision, recall, and F-measure. This model showed perfect accuracy on untagged features and achieved precision levels of 98.9% for the CKD data and 95.9% for the Hungarian data.

The research by V S Pavan Kumar et al. (Pavan Kumar et al., 2025) developed a high-accuracy diagnosis system for CKD through three primary approaches: feature selection, ensemble modeling, and data preprocessing stages. The BFO acts as a feature selector to maximize model efficiency through its accuracy enhancement of a more compact predictive model by noticing both blood pressure and albumin level importance during feature elimination. The data set receives preprocessing through IQR method outlier treatment to address outliers and the SMOTE method to manage class imbalance problems, which ensures high-quality data set input.

3. CONCLUSION

DNN systems, when merged with clinical data and medical imaging, have promising capabilities to improve early CKD detection and prediction. Hospital patients can achieve complete health assessments by integrating medical imaging data with laboratory results and patient medical histories. The combination of DNN models, particularly convolutional neural networks (CNNs), enables better prediction accuracy when processing image- and non-image-based input. Additional challenges remain in the way of successful implementation due to the necessity of considerable dataset quantities, data balancing, and model interpretability, which are essential for clinical use scenarios. The next phase of research will work to enhance model clarity while handling actual clinical restrictions and creating combinations of DNN systems with other AI methods. Future implementation of cutting-edge medical methods requires standardized frameworks and better data processing systems because they enable successful use across different healthcare environments. This conclusion demonstrates that DNNs will transform CKD prediction and provide essential knowledge about clinical research and system innovation.

REFERENCES

Akhtar, M. N., Iqbal, M. K., & Abid, M. S. (2025). Renal vision advanced kidney disease detection using attention-powered ensemble CNNs. Physical Education. *Health and Social Sciences*, *3*(1), 31–42.

Akter, S., Habib, A., Islam, M. A., Hossen, M. S., Fahim, W. A., Sarkar, P. R., & Ahmed, M. (2021). Comprehensive performance assessment of deep learning models in early prediction and risk identification of chronic kidney disease. *IEEE Access : Practical Innovations, Open Solutions*, *9*, 165184–165206. DOI: 10.1109/ACCESS.2021.3134130

Alalawi, H. H., & Alsuwat, M. S. (2021). Detection of cardiovascular disease using machine learning classification models. *International Journal of Engineering Research & Technology (Ahmedabad)*, *10*(7), 151–157.

Alikhan, J. S., Alageswaran, R., & Miruna Joe Amali, S. (2023). Self-attention convolutional neural network optimized with season optimization algorithm espoused chronic kidney diseases diagnosis in big data system. *Biomedical Signal Processing and Control*, *85*, 105011. Advance online publication. DOI: 10.1016/j.bspc.2023.105011

Almustafa, K. M. (2021). Prediction of chronic kidney disease using different classification algorithms. *Informatics in Medicine Unlocked*, *24*, 100631. Advance online publication. DOI: 10.1016/j.imu.2021.100631

Antony, L., Azam, S., Ignatious, E., Quadir, R., Beeravolu, A. R., Jonkman, M., & De Boer, F. (2021). A comprehensive unsupervised framework for chronic kidney disease prediction. *IEEE Access : Practical Innovations, Open Solutions*, *9*, 126481–126501. DOI: 10.1109/ACCESS.2021.3109168

Aprilianto, D. (2020). SVM optimization with correlation feature selection based binary particle swarm optimization for diagnosis of chronic kidney disease. *Journal of Soft Computing Exploration*, *1*(1), 24–31.

Baghdadi, N. A., Farghaly Abdelaliem, S. M., Malki, A., Gad, I., Ewis, A., & Atlam, E.-S. (2023). Advanced machine learning techniques for cardiovascular disease early detection and diagnosis. *Journal of Big Data*, *10*(1), 144. Advance online publication. DOI: 10.1186/s40537-023-00814-8

Bai, Q., Su, C., Tang, W., & Li, Y. (2022). Machine learning to predict end stage kidney disease in chronic kidney disease. *Scientific Reports*, *12*(1), 8377. Advance online publication. DOI: 10.1038/s41598-022-11757-6 PMID: 35589908

Bhak, Y., Lee, Y. H., Kim, J., Lee, K., Lee, D., Jang, E. C., & Jang, E. (2025). Diagnosis of chronic kidney disease using retinal imaging and urine dipstick data: Multimodal deep learning approach. *JMIR Medical Informatics*, *13*(1), e55825. PMID: 39924305

Burra, L. R., Tumuluru, P., Bonam, J., Raju, S. H., Nalajala, S., & Borra, S. P. R. (2025). Innovative application of conditional deep convolutional generative adversarial networks to enhance chronic kidney disease diagnosis with uneven datasets. In Smart factories for Industry 5.0 transformation (pp. 71–87).

Chandralekha, E., Vinodhini, S., Kandasamy, V., Rama, P., Ravikumar, S., & Saravanan, T. R. (2023). An extensive machine learning framework employing ensemble classifiers for heart disease detection. In 2023 3rd International Conference on Innovative Mechanisms for Industry Applications (ICIMIA) (pp. 973–978). IEEE. https://doi.org/DOI: 10.1109/ICIMIA60397.2023.10084912

Chang, Y.-J., Lin, C.-H., & Chien, Y.-C. (2025). Predicting the risk of chronic kidney disease based on uric acid concentration in stones using biosensors integrated with a deep learning-based ANN system. *Talanta*, *283*, 127077. PMID: 39476796

Debal, D. A., & Sitote, T. M. (2022). Chronic kidney disease prediction using machine learning techniques. *Journal of Big Data*, *9*(1), 109. Advance online publication. DOI: 10.1186/s40537-022-00657-5

Ferguson, T., Ravani, P., Sood, M. M., Clarke, A., Komenda, P., Rigatto, C., & Tangri, N. (2022). Development and external validation of a machine learning model for progression of CKD. *Kidney International Reports*, *7*(8), 1772–1781. DOI: 10.1016/j.ekir.2022.05.028 PMID: 35967110

Geng, T.-T., Chen, J.-X., Lu, Q., Wang, P.-L., Xia, P.-F., Zhu, K., & Li, Y. (2024). Nuclear magnetic resonance–based metabolomics and risk of CKD. *American Journal of Kidney Diseases*, *83*(1), 9–17. DOI: 10.1053/j.ajkd.2023.06.007 PMID: 37678743

George, C., Echouffo-Tcheugui, J. B., Jaar, B. G., Okpechi, I. G., & Kengne, A. P. (2022). The need for screening, early diagnosis, and prediction of chronic kidney disease in people with diabetes in low- and middle-income countries—A review of the current literature. *BMC Medicine*, *20*(1), 247. Advance online publication. DOI: 10.1186/s12916-022-02466-5 PMID: 35915501

Iftikhar, H., Khan, M., Khan, Z., Khan, F., Alshanbari, H. M., & Ahmad, Z. (2023). A comparative analysis of machine learning models: A case study in predicting chronic kidney disease. *Sustainability*, *15*(3), 2754. Advance online publication. DOI: 10.3390/su15032754

Iliyas, I. I., Isa, A., Zarma, M. L., & Dauda, B. A. (2025). Deep learning in predicting genetic disorders: A case study of diabetic kidney disease. In *Deep learning in genetics and genomics* (pp. 329–347). Academic Press.

Iqbal, S., Qureshi, A. N., Alhussein, M., Aurangzeb, K., Zubair, M., & Hussain, A. (2025). A novel reciprocal domain adaptation neural network for enhanced diagnosis of chronic kidney disease. *Expert Systems: International Journal of Knowledge Engineering and Neural Networks*, *42*(2), e13825.

Islam, M. A., Majumder, M. Z. H., & Hussein, M. A. (2023). Chronic kidney disease prediction based on machine learning algorithms. *Journal of Pathology Informatics*, *14*, 100189. Advance online publication. DOI: 10.1016/j.jpi.2023.100189 PMID: 36714452

Ismail, W. N. (2023). Snake-efficient feature selection-based framework for precise early detection of chronic kidney disease. *Diagnostics (Basel)*, *13*(15), 2501. Advance online publication. DOI: 10.3390/diagnostics13152501 PMID: 37568865

Jabbar, F. A., & Rithanya, K. S. (2021). Risks of chronic kidney disease prediction using various data mining algorithms. International Journal of Informatics [INJIIS-COM]. *Information System and Computer Engineering*, *2*(2), 165–177.

Jacquline, M. L., & Sudha, N. (2024). Chronic kidney disease classification using entropy based butterfly optimization and improved artificial neural network algorithm: Preprocessing, feature selection, clustering, and disease prediction. *Journal of Angiotherapy*, *8*(6), 1–12.

Jerlin Rubini, L., & Perumal, E. (2020). Efficient classification of chronic kidney disease by using multi-kernel support vector machine and fruit fly optimization algorithm. *International Journal of Imaging Systems and Technology*, *30*(3), 660–673. DOI: 10.1002/ima.22406

Jerlin Rubini, L., & Perumal, E. (2022). Oppositional firefly optimization based optimal feature selection in chronic kidney disease classification using deep neural network. *Journal of Ambient Intelligence and Humanized Computing*, *13*(4), 1799–1810. DOI: 10.1007/s12652-020-02824-5

Khalid, H., Khan, A., Khan, M. Z., Mehmood, G., & Qureshi, M. S. (2023). Machine learning hybrid model for the prediction of chronic kidney disease. *Computational Intelligence and Neuroscience*, *2023*, 9266889. Advance online publication. DOI: 10.1155/2023/9266889 PMID: 36959840

Kumari, S., & Singh, S. K. (2022). An ensemble learning-based model for effective chronic kidney disease prediction. In *2022 International Conference on Computing, Communication, and Intelligent Systems (ICCCIS)* (pp. 162–168). IEEE. https://doi .org/DOI: 10.1109/ICCCIS56430.2022.10037562

Lakshmi, K. L., Umadevi, M., & Bellamkonda, L. P. (2025). Optimized truncated singular value decomposition and hybrid deep neural network with random forest for automated disease prediction. *Biomedical Signal Processing and Control, 100*, 107010.

Ma, J., Wang, J., Lu, L., Sun, Y., Feng, M., Shen, P., Jiang, Z., Hong, S., & Zhang, L. (2025). Development and validation of a dynamic kidney failure prediction model based on deep learning: A real-world study with external validation. arXiv preprint arXiv:2501.16388.

Mandula, A., & Vijaya Kumar, B. S. (2024). Integrated feature selection and ensemble learning for heart disease detection: A 2-tier approach with ALAN and ET-ABDF machine learning model. *International Journal of Information Technology : an Official Journal of Bharati Vidyapeeth's Institute of Computer Applications and Management*, *16*(7), 4489–4503. DOI: 10.1007/s41870-024-02245-6

Mehta, V., Batra, N., Goyal, S., Kaur, A., Dudekula, K. V., & Victor, G. J. (2024). Machine Learning based Exploratory Data Analysis (EDA) and Diagnosis of Chronic Kidney Disease (CKD). *EAI Endorsed Transactions on Pervasive Health and Technology*, *10*(1), e4.

Mittal, P., Sharma, Y. K., Lilhore, U. K., Simaiya, S., Saleem, K., & Ghith, E. S. (2025). Advanced Hybrid Machine Learning Model for Accurate Detection of Cardiovascular Disease. *International Journal of Computational Intelligence Systems*, *18*(1), 1–20.

Pal, S. (2023). Chronic kidney disease prediction using machine learning techniques. *Biomedical Materials & Devices*, *1*, 534–540. DOI: 10.1007/s44174-022-00027-y

Pavan Kumar, V. S., Yadla, J., Parvatham, N. K., Lokesh Kumar, P., Tulluri, U., & Amrutha, K. (2025). Optimized predictive modelling for chronic kidney disease: A hybrid ensemble approach with bacterial foraging optimization and SMOTE. In 2025 6th International Conference on Mobile Computing and Sustainable Informatics (ICMCSI) (pp. 988–994). IEEE.

Pradeepa, P., & Jeyakumar, M. K. (2024). Chronic kidney disease prediction using improved deep belief network with local search nearest neighbour optimization. *Computer Methods in Biomechanics and Biomedical Engineering. Imaging & Visualization*, *11*(7), 2292085. Advance online publication. DOI: 10.1080/21681163.2024.2292085

Praveen, S. P., Jyothi, V. E., Anuradha, C., Venugopal, K., Shariff, V., & Sindhura, S. (2024). Chronic kidney disease prediction using ML-based Neuro-Fuzzy model. *International Journal of Image and Graphics*, *24*(6), 2340013. Advance online publication. DOI: 10.1142/S021946782340013X

Ramspek, C. L., Evans, M., Wanner, C., Drechsler, C., Chesnaye, N. C., Szymczak, M., & Krajewska, M.EQUAL Study Investigators. (2021). Kidney failure prediction models: A comprehensive external validation study in patients with advanced CKD. *Journal of the American Society of Nephrology*, *32*(5), 1174–1186. DOI: 10.1681/ASN.2020071077 PMID: 33685974

Ramu, K., Patthi, S., Prajapati, Y. N., Ramesh, J. V. N., Banerjee, S., Brahma Rao, K. B. V., & Alzahrani, S. I. (2025). Hybrid CNN-SVM model for enhanced early detection of chronic kidney disease. *Biomedical Signal Processing and Control*, *100*, 107084. Advance online publication. DOI: 10.1016/j.bspc.2024.107084

Rashed-Al-Mahfuz, M., Haque, A., Azad, A., Alyami, S. A., Quinn, J. M. W., & Moni, M. A. (2021). Clinically applicable machine learning approaches to identify attributes of chronic kidney disease (CKD) for use in low-cost diagnostic screening. *IEEE Journal of Translational Engineering in Health and Medicine*, *9*, 1–11. DOI: 10.1109/JTEHM.2021.3073629 PMID: 33948393

Rath, A., Mishra, D., & Panda, G. (2021). LSTM-based cardiovascular disease detection using ECG signal. In Cognitive informatics and soft computing: Proceedings of CISC 2020 (pp. 133–142). Springer Singapore. https://doi.org/DOI: 10.1007/978-981-16-1056-1_12

Rubini, L. J., & Perumal, E. (2020). Hybrid kernel support vector machine classifier and grey wolf optimization algorithm based intelligent classification algorithm for chronic kidney disease. *Journal of Medical Imaging and Health Informatics*, *10*(10), 2297–2307. DOI: 10.1166/jmihi.2020.3192

Sara, S. B. V. J., & Kalaiselvi, K. (2019). Ant colony optimization (ACO) based feature selection and extreme learning machine (ELM) for chronic kidney disease detection. *International Journal of Advanced Studies of Scientific Research*, *4*(1).

Sawhney, R., Malik, A., Sharma, S., & Narayan, V. (2023). A comparative assessment of artificial intelligence models used for early prediction and evaluation of chronic kidney disease. *Decision Analytics Journal*, *6*, 100169. Advance online publication. DOI: 10.1016/j.dajour.2023.100169

Shorewala, V. (2021). Early detection of coronary heart disease using ensemble techniques. *Informatics in Medicine Unlocked*, *26*, 100655. Advance online publication. DOI: 10.1016/j.imu.2021.100655

Sitaraman, S. R., Alagarsundaram, P., Gattupalli, K., Gollavilli, V. S. B. H., Nagarajan, H., & Ajao, L. A. (2024). Advanced IoMT-enabled chronic kidney disease prediction leveraging robotic automation with autoencoder-LSTM and fuzzy cognitive maps. *International Journal of Modern Electronics and Communication Engineering*, *12*(3), 1–20.

Subasi, A., Alickovic, E., & Kevric, J. (2017). Diagnosis of chronic kidney disease by using random forest. In CMBEBIH 2017: Proceedings of the International Conference on Medical and Biological Engineering 2017 (pp. 589–594). Springer Singapore. https://doi.org/DOI: 10.1007/978-981-10-4166-2_89

Terrada, O., Hamida, S., Cherradi, B., Raihani, A., & Bouattane, O. (2020). Supervised machine learning based medical diagnosis support system for prediction of patients with heart disease. *Advances in Science, Technology and Engineering Systems Journal*, *5*(5), 269–277. DOI: 10.25046/aj050534

Van Slobbe, R., Herrmannova, D., Boeke, D. J., Lima-Walton, E. S., Abu-Hanna, A., & Vagliano, I. (2025). Multimodal convolutional neural networks for the prediction of acute kidney injury in the intensive care. *International Journal of Medical Informatics*, •••, 105815. PMID: 39914070

Yewale, D., Vijayaragavan, S. P., & Bairagi, V. K. (2023). An effective heart disease prediction framework based on ensemble techniques in machine learning. *International Journal of Advanced Computer Science and Applications*, *14*(2), 1–10.

Chapter 7
Evaluating VGG16, ResNet50, and Xception for COVID-19 Detection via a Web-Based Deep Learning Interface

Snehal Rahul Rathi
https://orcid.org/0009-0004-7638-6429
Vishwakarma Institute of Technology, Pune, India

Chitra Joshi
Vishwakarma Institute of Information Technology, Pune, India

Atharva Pardeshi
Vishwakarma Institute of Information Technology, Pune, India

Anushka Bhagwat
Vishwakarma Institute of Information Technology, Pune, India

ABSTRACT

The global outbreak of COVID-19 has emphasized the need for fast and accurate diagnostic methods, especially in areas where advanced testing facilities are scarce or unavailable. This research proposes a deep learning-based method for the binary classification of chest X-ray images aimed at detecting COVID-19 infections. We evaluate and compare the performance of three prominent Convolutional Neural Network (CNN) architectures ResNet50, VGG16, and Xception trained on publicly available chest radiograph datasets. Additionally, a confusion matrix, training versus

DOI: 10.4018/979-8-3373-0179-2.ch007

ht © 2026, IGI Global Scientific Publishing. Copying or distributing in print or electronic forms without written permission of IGI Global Scientific Publishing is prohibited. Use of this chapter to generative artificial intelligence (AI) technologies is expressly prohibited. The publisher reserves all rights to license its use for generative AI training and machine learning model development.

validation accuracy plots, and the ROC curve are employed to gain deeper insights into the model's effectiveness and diagnostic capability. To enhance usability, a user-friendly web interface has also been developed, enabling users to upload images and obtain real-time classification results. Experimental findings indicate that all three models perform well in distinguishing COVID-19 cases, with the Xception model achieving the highest accuracy.

I. INTRODUCTION

COVID-19 created a worldwide public health emergency and as a result there was urgent need for cost-efficient, reliable, and scalable ways of diagnosing patients with this disease and the rest of the population as well. RT-PCR (Reverse Transcriptase-Polymerase Chain Reaction Testing) is currently regarded as the gold standard diagnostic test for diagnosing COVID-19. However, RT-PCR has many limitations, such as being expensive, having limited access to patients, and providing a delay in obtaining results.

The application of Deep Learning, particularly Convolutional Neural Networks (CNNs), to automated medical image analysis, has made significant advances in the ability of medical professionals to quickly identify patterns in large amounts of medical images. CNNs learn the features of a medical image just from the pixels of the image. CNN's ability to learn the image features has made it possible for medical professionals to use them to classify images into many categories. It has been demonstrated that several types of pre-trained CNN networks have a high degree of accuracy when classifying images in many types of classification tasks, including medical diagnostic images. Many of the CNN networks use Transfer Learning methodology, whereby large data sets of typical images are used to train the models, and then they have been successfully adapted for much smaller medical imaging sets.

In this study we have investigated three widely used CNN architectures to perform binary classification tasks on chest X-rays by identifying COVID-19 positive cases from COVID-19 negative cases. Additionally, a web-based application developed using Django has been created for easy upload of chest X-ray images by health care workers or researchers and to receive instant diagnostic results for their uploaded chest X-ray images. Incorporating trained deep neural networks into a web server backend facilitates the efficient completion of inference and reporting results.

The primary goals of this work are:

1. To evaluate and compare the classification accuracies of three commonly used CNN architectures for detecting COVID-19; and

2. To create an interactive clinical decision-support tool that allows the end-user to convert the output of a trained model into a user-friendly format.

The combination of performance analysis and deployment of an application provides valuable contributions to the body of knowledge relating to the use of artificial intelligence in healthcare and illustrates the practicality of using chest X-rays for real-time detection of COVID-19.

II. EASE OF USE

The system has been developed for usability with easy access to the application for all users, irrespective of how familiar they may be with the technical aspects of the application. Users can interact smoothly with the web interface, designed with Django as the backend and HTML, CSS, and Bootstrap as the frontend, which allows for quick response times regardless of the user's device, platform, or connection speed.

After uploading the chest X-ray image from their own device, the users need to simply click the "Solve" button and the backend will utilize all three pre-trained CNN models - ResNet50, VGG16, and Xception, which will return a prediction associated with the chest X-ray image after performing processing on the backend (Gururaj et al., 2024). The results will be displayed in a neatly laid out table format that shows comparisons of the predictions side by side.

The application's user interface was designed to look attractive, provide an easy and intuitive way for a user to interact with the system, and support rapid interaction with the system, all without the need for the user to possess any advanced technical skills. The main page of the application has bright colours, which provide a colourful background, and an eye-catching display of the application's title "COV-CNN" across the top of the application.

Within the centre of the page, is the file uploader, which contains:

- A button, referred to as "Choose File", that allows a user to open their own file system to select a chest X-ray image to upload.
- A button, referred to as "Solve", that can be pressed to initiate the backend processing and return the final prediction from the three different CNN models.

Figure 1. Overview of the Final Outcome

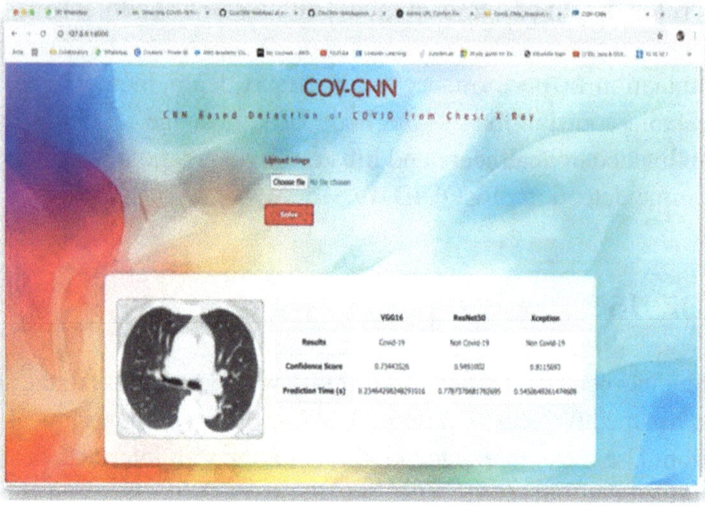

Once an image is uploaded and processed, the results are displayed in a well-organized layout:

- On the **left**, the uploaded chest X-ray image is shown.
- On the **right**, a **results table** is presented with columns for each model—**VGG16**, **ResNet50**, and **Xception**.

- The table includes three rows:

- **Results** – indicating whether each model classified the image as "COVID-19" or "Normal".
- **Confidence Score** – showing the model's confidence in its prediction.
- **Prediction Time (s)** – detailing the time taken by each model to generate its result.

This side-by-side comparison in a compact table provides users with a quick overview of model agreement and performance, enhancing interpretability and trust in the system's predictions.

III. LITERATURE REVIEW

Although RT-PCR tests remain the most commonly used formal method for diagnosing COVID-19, these tests can take time for the results, they can be expensive, and not everyone can get access to them for various reasons. A quicker alternative to RT-PCR tests are Chest X-rays however they must be read manually which means you must have a certain level of medical expertise and there is always a potential for error. This research project has developed a method of automatically reading Chest X-rays for detection of COVID-19 using deep learning techniques in particular the use of three separate convolutional neural networks (CNN) — VGG16, ResNet50, and Xception — to enable comparison of the performance of the models and also allow for real time diagnosis through the use of a web-based platform to display the results.

Asif et al. (2020) developed a CNN that was able to extract significant visual characteristics from CXR images of COVID-19 patients and were able to achieve over 90% accuracy on their test set, this demonstrates the capability of CNNs to reliably identify COVID-19 related defects in Radiological Imaging. Heidari et al., 2020 improved on the performance of CNNs by including software programs that perform pre-processing techniques including removing noise and improving contrast from CXR images. The pre-processing techniques considerably increased the performance of their model as this demonstrates the critical role that the data analysis process plays in the effectiveness of the analysis of Medical Imaging.

Abbas et al. (2021) introduced a model named DeTraC which uses Class Decomposition to improve on the performance of CNNs when confronted with irregular and imbalanced data sets. The use of class decomposition resulted in the development of more precise boundaries between each class thus improving the accuracy of the models. Hussain et al. (2021) proposed the CoroDet, which is a new CNN architecture for COVID-19 detection. By utilising model tuning and normalisation of the dataset, they were able to achieve an exceptional 95% accurate classification.

Dynamic CNN architecture capable of modifying its structural framework (including the ability to combine CXR and CT image classification) for better COVID-19 classification was developed by Jia et al., 2021. Their results show strong classification ability to discriminate between COVID-19 and other lower respiratory conditions, reflecting a high adaptability of their models.

Dasare and H.S. (2021) proposed a CNN-based classification system for COVID-19 detection with minimal input data. Their results illustrate that even with minimal training data, CNNs produce robust classification performance, making it a very suitable model for real-time, scalable distribution.

Lastly, Gururaj et al. (2024) reported on high-level trends in CNN-based systems for the diagnosis of COVID-19 as part of a broader investigation into the development of intelligent healthcare systems. The findings in this report provide insight into the increasing impact of AI on improved healthcare delivery systems, particularly during Pandemic times.

IV. RESEARCH METHODOLOGY

The whole system is made to provide a web-based interface for simplicity of access and use. The main elements of the approach are enumerated here:

A. Dataset Description

Aiming for this work, we used the freely available medical imaging dataset kept on Kaggle (de Moura, 2021; Ibrahim et al., 2021). This dataset consists of CT scan images taken from real-world patients.

Capturing cross-sectional views of the lungs, this dataset is a carefully chosen collection of CT scan images rather than X-rays. It comprises images falling into two categories:

- Positive COVID-19 (SARS-CoV-2 infected lungs)
- Negative for COVID-19 (either healthy or non-COVID lung scans)

B. Implementation

Three pre-trained CNN models are used as follows:

1. **VGG16**: a 16-layer classic deep CNN model distinguished by its simple design and homogeneous architecture. For general-purpose classification chores and transfer learning, it performs well.

   Architecture Highlights:

   - **Convolutional Layers**: VGG16 uses **13 convolutional layers**, all with small **3×3 filters**, stride 1, and padding to preserve spatial resolution. This consistent kernel size helps the network capture fine details in the images.
   - **Fully Connected Layers**: The final part of the network includes **three dense layers** (two with 4096 units and one output layer), acting as classifiers after feature extraction.
   - **ReLU Activation**: All layers use the **ReLU** activation function, enabling faster training and preventing vanishing gradients.

Figure 2. Model Summary - VGG16

Model: "functional_1"

Layer (type)	Output Shape	Param #
input_layer_1 (InputLayer)	(None, 150, 150, 3)	0
block1_conv1 (Conv2D)	(None, 150, 150, 64)	1,792
block1_conv2 (Conv2D)	(None, 150, 150, 64)	36,928
block1_pool (MaxPooling2D)	(None, 75, 75, 64)	0
block2_conv1 (Conv2D)	(None, 75, 75, 128)	73,856
block2_conv2 (Conv2D)	(None, 75, 75, 128)	147,584
block2_pool (MaxPooling2D)	(None, 37, 37, 128)	0
block3_conv1 (Conv2D)	(None, 37, 37, 256)	295,168
block3_conv2 (Conv2D)	(None, 37, 37, 256)	590,080
block3_conv3 (Conv2D)	(None, 37, 37, 256)	590,080
block3_pool (MaxPooling2D)	(None, 18, 18, 256)	0
block4_conv1 (Conv2D)	(None, 18, 18, 512)	1,180,160
block4_conv2 (Conv2D)	(None, 18, 18, 512)	2,359,808
block4_conv3 (Conv2D)	(None, 18, 18, 512)	2,359,808
block4_pool (MaxPooling2D)	(None, 9, 9, 512)	0
block5_conv1 (Conv2D)	(None, 9, 9, 512)	2,359,808
block5_conv2 (Conv2D)	(None, 9, 9, 512)	2,359,808
block5_conv3 (Conv2D)	(None, 9, 9, 512)	2,359,808
block5_pool (MaxPooling2D)	(None, 4, 4, 512)	0
global_average_pooling2d_1 (GlobalAveragePooling2D)	(None, 512)	0
batch_normalization_2 (BatchNormalization)	(None, 512)	2,048
dropout_2 (Dropout)	(None, 512)	0
dense_2 (Dense)	(None, 256)	131,328
batch_normalization_3 (BatchNormalization)	(None, 256)	1,024
dropout_3 (Dropout)	(None, 256)	0
dense_3 (Dense)	(None, 2)	514

Total params: 14,849,602 (56.65 MB)
Trainable params: 133,378 (521.01 KB)
Non-trainable params: 14,716,224 (56.14 MB)

Figure 3. System Architecture - VGG16

Model: "functional_1"

Layer (type)	Output Shape	Param #
input_layer_1 (InputLayer)	(None, 150, 150, 3)	0
block1_conv1 (Conv2D)	(None, 150, 150, 64)	1,792
block1_conv2 (Conv2D)	(None, 150, 150, 64)	36,928
block1_pool (MaxPooling2D)	(None, 75, 75, 64)	0
block2_conv1 (Conv2D)	(None, 75, 75, 128)	73,856
block2_conv2 (Conv2D)	(None, 75, 75, 128)	147,584
block2_pool (MaxPooling2D)	(None, 37, 37, 128)	0
block3_conv1 (Conv2D)	(None, 37, 37, 256)	295,168
block3_conv2 (Conv2D)	(None, 37, 37, 256)	590,080
block3_conv3 (Conv2D)	(None, 37, 37, 256)	590,080
block3_pool (MaxPooling2D)	(None, 18, 18, 256)	0
block4_conv1 (Conv2D)	(None, 18, 18, 512)	1,180,160
block4_conv2 (Conv2D)	(None, 18, 18, 512)	2,359,808
block4_conv3 (Conv2D)	(None, 18, 18, 512)	2,359,808
block4_pool (MaxPooling2D)	(None, 9, 9, 512)	0
block5_conv1 (Conv2D)	(None, 9, 9, 512)	2,359,808
block5_conv2 (Conv2D)	(None, 9, 9, 512)	2,359,808
block5_conv3 (Conv2D)	(None, 9, 9, 512)	2,359,808
block5_pool (MaxPooling2D)	(None, 4, 4, 512)	0
global_average_pooling2d_1 (GlobalAveragePooling2D)	(None, 512)	0
batch_normalization_2 (BatchNormalization)	(None, 512)	2,048
dropout_2 (Dropout)	(None, 512)	0
dense_2 (Dense)	(None, 256)	131,328
batch_normalization_3 (BatchNormalization)	(None, 256)	1,024
dropout_3 (Dropout)	(None, 256)	0
dense_3 (Dense)	(None, 2)	514

Total params: 14,849,602 (56.65 MB)
Trainable params: 133,378 (521.01 KB)
Non-trainable params: 14,716,224 (56.14 MB)

Why VGG16 is Useful in This Study: VGG16 has been found to be a useful tool during this research. Due to its complexity and number of layers (16), along with using transfer learning using a medical image dataset, it will create a strong baseline model for feature extraction from the medical images.

2. **ResNet50**: ResNet50 is a deep CNN model created by Microsoft Research with 50 layers. It allows for the training of extremely deep networks while avoiding problems related to degradation in performance as the number of layers increases. ResNet50 is part of the Residual Network (ResNet) family, which is built upon the foundation of addressing the vanishing gradient issue using skip connections, also called residual blocks, to make gradients flow more easily through the various layers. This results in better training of very deep neural networks.

   Architecture Highlights:

   - **Residual Blocks**: The main advancement of ResNet50 is through the use of residual blocks with skip connections. These allow for resolving problems associated with very deep neural networks such as degradation or vanishing gradients.

- **Batch Normalization**: After each convolution, batch normalization is applied to stabilize and accelerate training.
- **50 Layers**: ResNet50 has a total of 50 layers, making it substantially deeper than VGG16 while remaining more straightforward to optimise than those without residual designs.
- **Weight Initialization**: ResNet architectures benefit greatly from pretrained weights (e.g., on ImageNet), which helps achieve high performance even with smaller datasets.

Figure 4. Model Summary - ResNet50

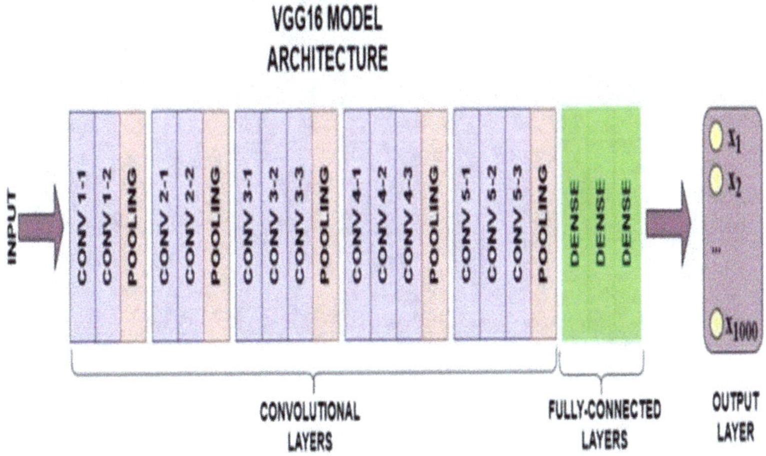

Why ResNet50 is Useful in This Study: Its deeper architecture and residual connections allow for more complex pattern recognition without degradation in performance, making it effective for subtle features in medical imaging.

Figure 5. System Architecture - ResNet50

Model: "functional_3"

Layer (type)	Output Shape	Param #
input_layer_7 (InputLayer)	(None, 64, 64, 3)	0
resnet50 (Functional)	(None, 2, 2, 2048)	23,587,712
global_average_pooling2d_3 (GlobalAveragePooling2D)	(None, 2048)	0
batch_normalization_6 (BatchNormalization)	(None, 2048)	8,192
dropout_6 (Dropout)	(None, 2048)	0
dense_3 (Dense)	(None, 256)	524,544
batch_normalization_7 (BatchNormalization)	(None, 256)	1,024
dropout_7 (Dropout)	(None, 256)	0
root (Dense)	(None, 2)	514

Total params: 24,121,986 (92.02 MB)
Trainable params: 24,064,258 (91.80 MB)
Non-trainable params: 57,728 (225.50 KB)

3. **Xception**: Xception, is an advanced CNN architecture that improves upon the Inception family.

Figure 6. System Architecture - Xception

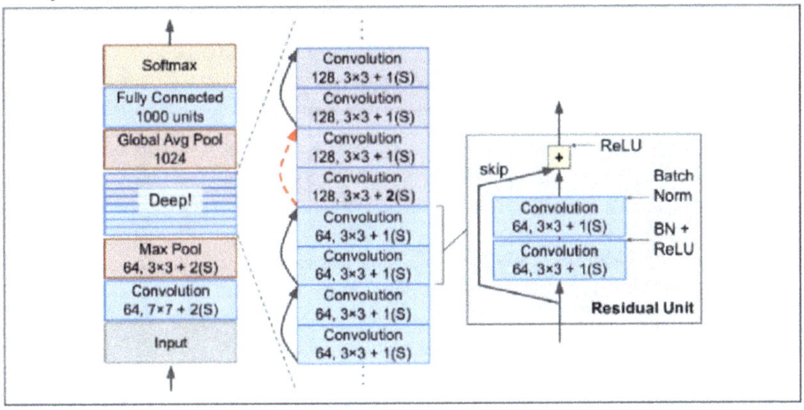

Architecture Highlights:

- **Entry, Middle, and Exit Flows**: The network is organized into three functional blocks:
    - o **Entry flow**: Performs initial down sampling
    - o **Middle flow**: Contains multiple identical modules with depth wise separable convolutions
    - o **Exit flow**: Final feature extraction and classification
- **ReLU and Batch Normalization**: ReLU activation and batch normalization are used extensively to maintain stability and performance.

Why Xception is Useful in This Study: It combines **efficiency and performance**, making it ideal for real-time inference in a web application and well-suited for CT scan classification. These models are fine-tuned with additional dense layers on top, tailored for binary classification (COVID-positive or COVID-negative).

Figure 7. Model Summary - Xception

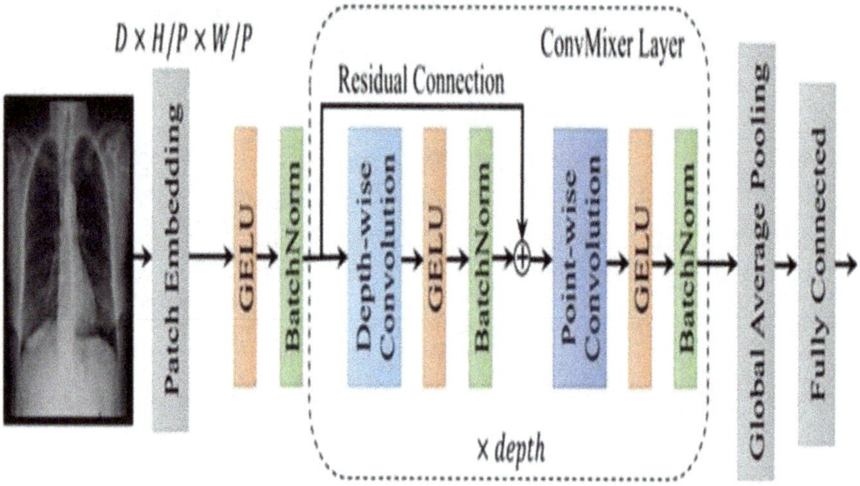

C. System Architecture and Workflow

System Architecture

The system has been created with an end-to-end pipeline that runs on a modular basis, combining machine learning predictions with web application capabilities in an uninterrupted stream of processing. The system architecture is divided into the following core elements:

User Interface (Frontend)

- Utilizing HTML, CSS and the Bootstrap framework.
- The front-end enables the user to submit a CT Chest scan for processing, creating a clean and simple layout for easy navigation of the results.
- The front-end submits the image to the back-end through a form.

Web Framework (Backend: Django)

- Django serves as the mediator between the front-end and the ML models.
- It is responsible for handling all HTTP requests, and managing files uploaded by users.
- It is also responsible for initiating and processing images in the classification pipeline and generating formatted and rendered results to the user using Django templates.

Model Layer (ML Inference Engine)

- Three pre-trained CNN models are loaded from TensorFlow using the Keras API.
- Each model independently processes the uploaded image and returns three outputs per model:
  1. COVID Status (Whether or Not the CT Scan Shows Signs of Infection)
  2. Probability Score (How Likely it is that the CT Scan Shows Signs of Infection)
  3. Time Taken for Each of the Models (How Long Each of the Models Took to Analyze the CT Scan)

Composite Results and Report

- The three results from each of the three models will be combined into one table.
- The table will show the predicted result from each model and the probability score and time required for each model to analyze the CT scan.
- The CT scan you uploaded will also be shown on the composite results page for your convenience.

Workflow

1. **Image Upload**
   - o The user selects a CT scan image and submits it through the web interface.
   - o The file is temporarily stored and sent to the backend for pre-processing.
2. **Image Pre-processing**
   - o Resizing of images was performed for the models to meet input requirements:
     - ▪ VGG16 and ResNet50: 224×224 pixels
     - ▪ Xception: 150×150 pixels
   - o Normalization is applied to scale pixel values to the [0,1] range.
   - o The image is reshaped to add the batch dimension expected by the model ((1, height, width, 3)).
3. **Model Inference**
   - o Each model loads its pre-trained weights (saved in .h5 format).
   - o The image is passed sequentially to all three models.
   - o Each model outputs:
     - ▪ Prediction class (0 or 1 → Negative or Positive)
     - ▪ SoftMax confidence score
     - ▪ Time Elapsed for making those predictions.
4. **Result Display**

- The processed output is rendered back on the same webpage.
- The user sees the uploaded image and a side-by-side comparison of the models' results.

D. Evaluation Metrics

The results of the models were evaluated using multiple metrics and metrics through a variety of visual methods. Evaluation of both the training and validation accuracy/loss graphs was performed to determine whether the models converged or overfitted during training. Additionally, a classification report created for each model with precision, recall, F1-Score, and support for each individual class provides an all-inclusive view of the performance of each model. To further analyze model predictions, confusion matrices and their visual representations (heat maps) were included to analyze how well the model was able to classify the results as accurate or inaccurate. Also, time taken by the model to produce an inference was calculated and compared against each model's computational efficiency. Together, these evaluation methods have provided a clear comparison of each of the three CNN models' diagnostic capabilities and resource trade-offs.

V. EXPERIMENTAL RESULTS

To do an extensive evaluation of the previously proposed deep-learning models for COVID-19 detection, we examined three different architectures (VGG16, ResNet50, and Xception) on their abilities to classify chest X-ray and CT scan images.

VGG16 is a very deep architecture (16 layers) and was found to achieve moderate performance (83% overall accuracy). For predicting COVID infection, the VGG16 model produced a reasonable F1-score of 0.85, but for predicting non-COVID infections, it only achieved a precision score of 0.77, which means that a number of non-COVID-pneumonia cases were miscategorized as positive.

The VGG16 model had a shorter inference time of about 0.85 seconds for each image, making it very efficient for rapid predictions, but lower accuracy and generalization at that speed. The confusion matrix showed that VGG16 correctly classified 120 out of 146 COVID positive cases and 87 out of 103 non-COVID positive cases, which resulted in a total of 26 false negative classifications and 16 false positive classifications. Thus, it is evident that this model mistakenly missed a portion of actual COVID positive cases. In light of this high rate of misclassification, it is less trustworthy for clinical applications, given its rapid inference time (~0.85 s/image).

Figure 8. Training(VGG16) vs Validation(VGG16) Accuracy

Model: "functional_1"

Layer (type)	Output Shape	Param #
input_layer_3 (InputLayer)	(None, 64, 64, 3)	0
conv2d_9 (Conv2D)	(None, 64, 64, 3)	84
xception (Functional)	(None, 2, 2, 2048)	20,861,480
global_average_pooling2d_1 (GlobalAveragePooling2D)	(None, 2048)	0
batch_normalization_10 (BatchNormalization)	(None, 2048)	8,192
dropout_2 (Dropout)	(None, 2048)	0
dense_1 (Dense)	(None, 256)	524,544
batch_normalization_11 (BatchNormalization)	(None, 256)	1,024
dropout_3 (Dropout)	(None, 256)	0
root (Dense)	(None, 2)	514

Total params: 21,395,838 (81.62 MB)
Trainable params: 21,336,702 (81.39 MB)
Non-trainable params: 59,136 (231.00 KB)

Figure 9. Training(VGG16) vs Validation(VGG16) Loss

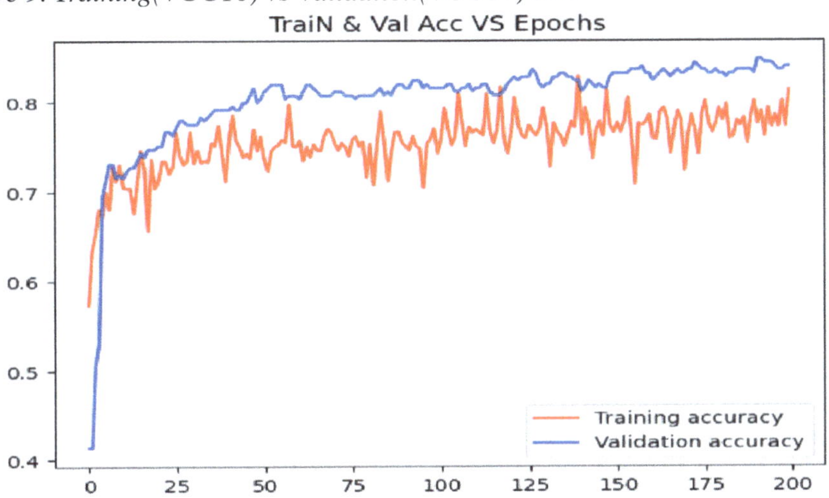

Figure 10. Confusion Matrix - VGG16

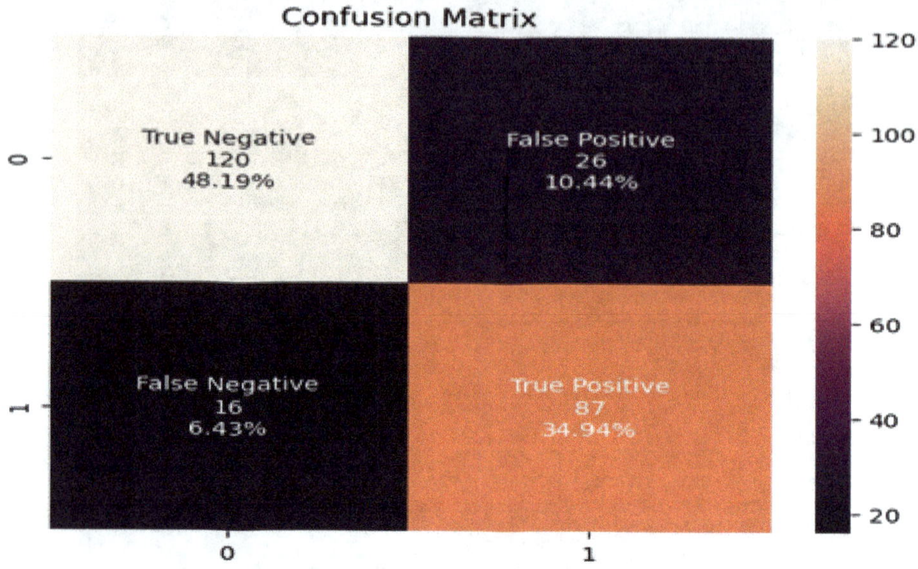

Figure 11. ROC Curve - VGG16

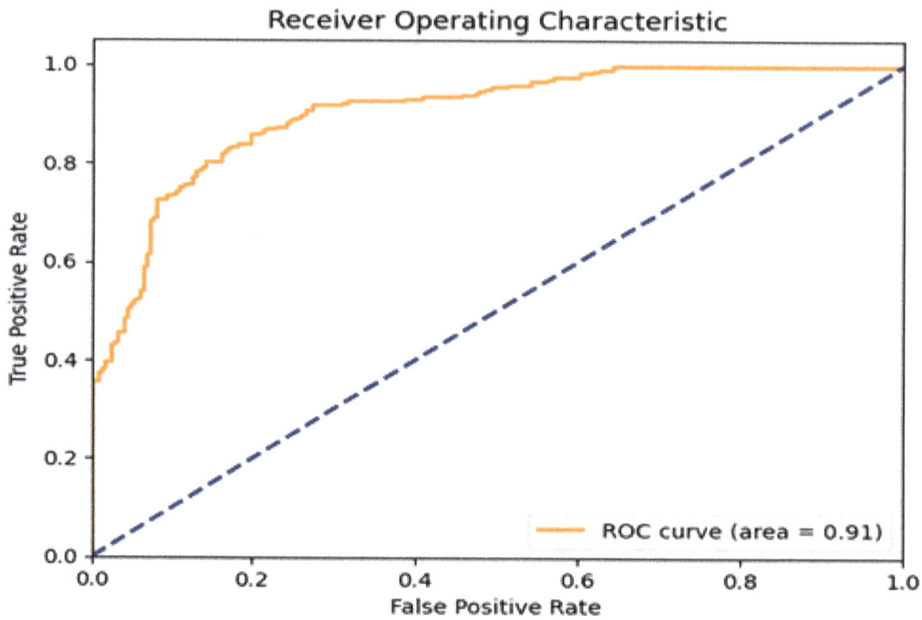

The ResNet50 architecture achieved overall superior performance on most evaluation metrics in comparison to VGG16. ResNet50's maximum validation accuracy was 88% and both of its f1 scores for classifying COVID and Non-COVID were 0.88, indicating balanced performance between classes. The tradeoff is that with greater accuracy, ResNet50 had more computational requirements and so it had a longer average inference time of ~1.12 seconds to process each image. In the confusion matrix, the ResNet50 correctly classified 218 of 243 actual COVID-19 positive instances and 222 of 255 actual Non-COVID-19 instances, indicating 25 false negatives and 33 false positives and providing evidence of improved generalization and robustness in comparison to VGG16. ResNet50's average time per image prediction was about 1.12 seconds. Although this average time was slightly longer, this increase in time is more than justified because of the increase in accuracy achieved by ResNet50.

Figure 12. Training(ResNet50) vs Validation(ResNet50) Accuracy

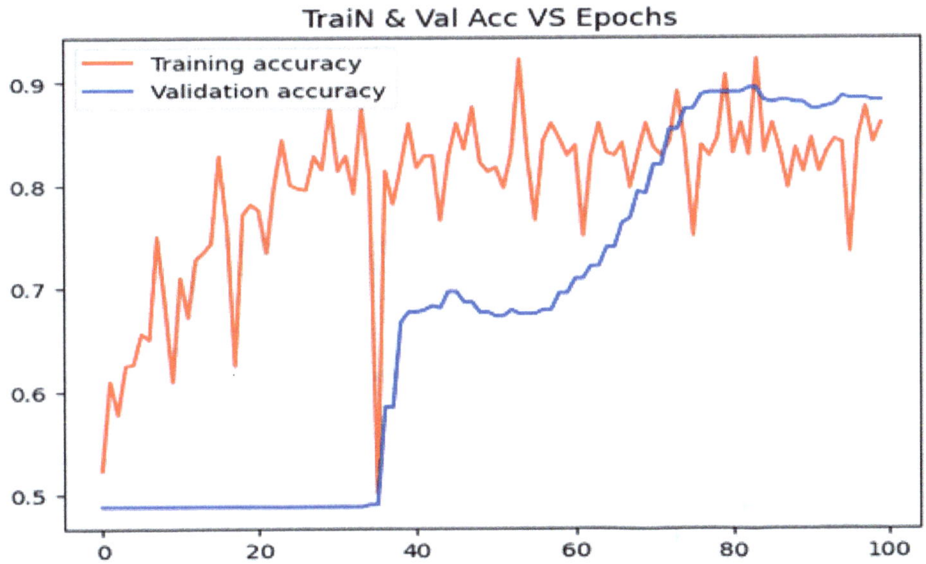

Figure 13. Training(ResNet50) vs Validation Loss(ResNet50)

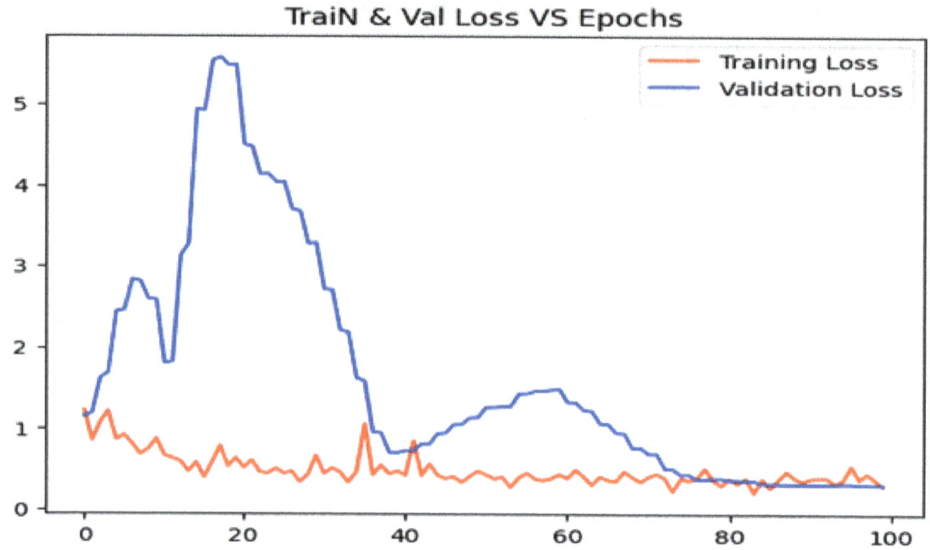

Figure 14. Confusion Matrix - ResNet50

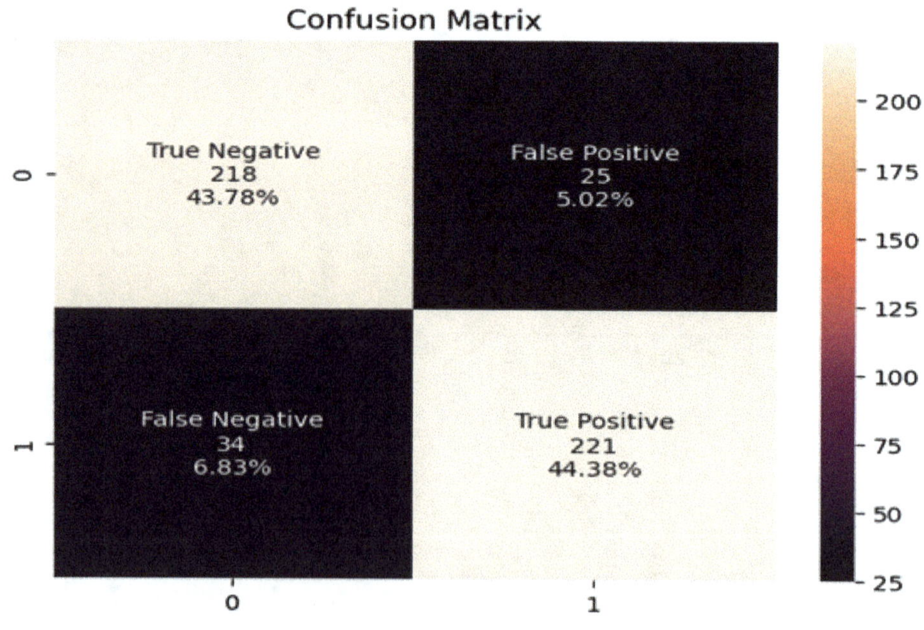

Figure 15. ROC Curve - ResNet50

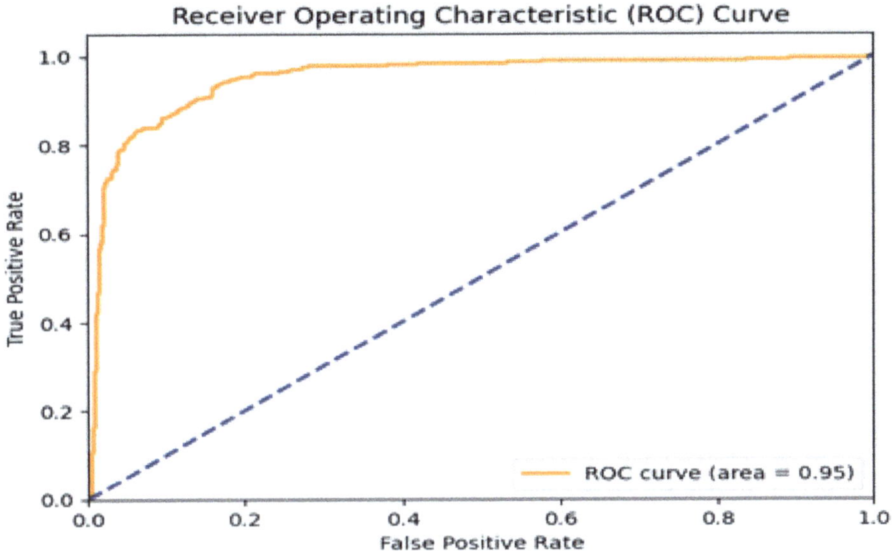

The newer and computationally efficient Xception model which employs depth wise separable convolutions also achieved 88 percent which is equal to ResNet50. The difference between the COVID and the non-COVID classes was quite small with F1-scores of 0.87 and 0.89 respectively. The Xception model did indeed make predictions faster than ResNet50 with approximately 0.95 seconds/image for inference. This shows that the Xception model well balances computational efficiency and predictive performance and is a contender for practical, time-sensitive settings. The confusion matrix shows that Xception accurately predicted 207 of 243 COVID cases and accurately predicted 232 of 255 non-COVID cases resulting in false negatives of 36 and false positives of 23. Although there were more false negatives for the Xception model than for the ResNet50 model, the inference of the Xception model at around 0.95 seconds/image is significantly faster than that of the ResNet50 model.

Figure 16. Training(Xception) vs Validation(Xception) Accuracy

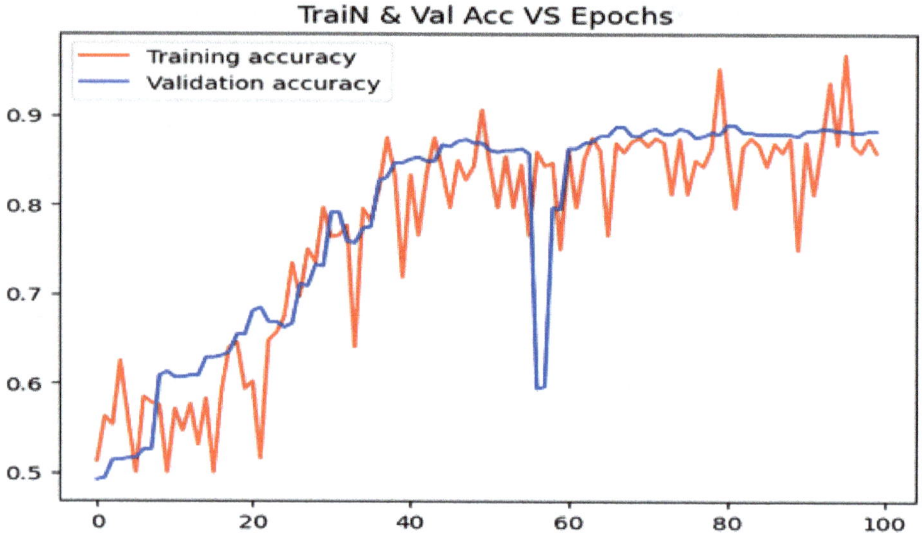

ResNet50 had slightly better classification accuracy than Xception but had a more balanced class classification while Xception had faster inference times compared to both VGG16 and ResNet50.

Figure 17. Training(Xception) vs Validation(Xception) Loss

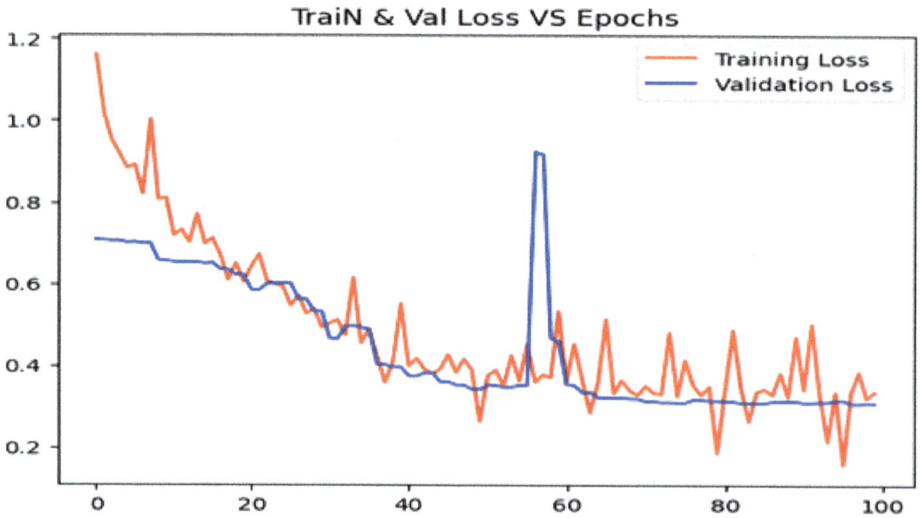

Figure 18. Confusion Matrix - Xception

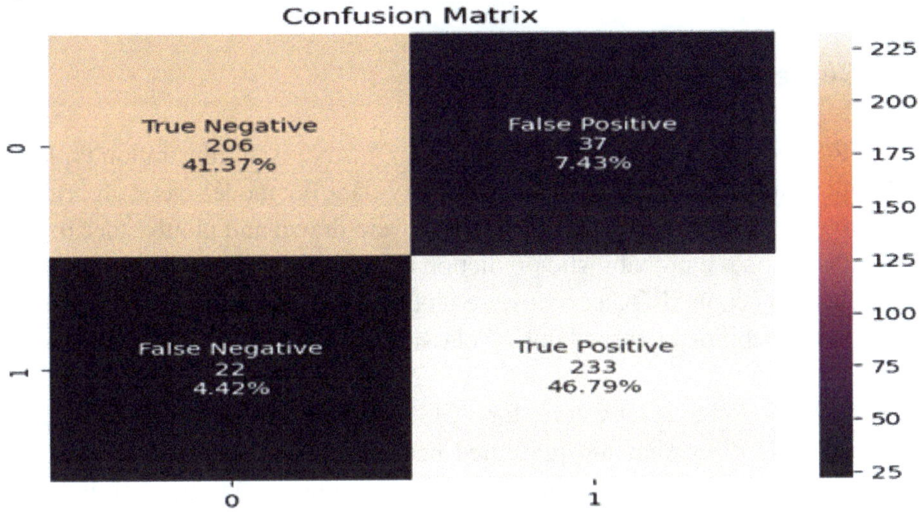

Figure 19. ROC Curve - Xception

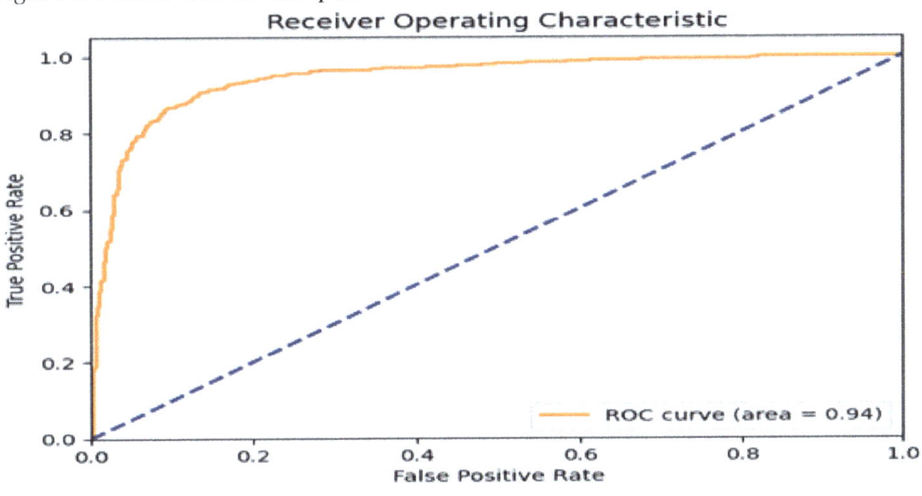

An analysis of the comparative results suggests that applicationspecific requirements, such as accuracyNeedsto be evaluated along with computational limits and latency, when selecting which model(s) will perform best. Our comparison study indicates that the most accurate models are ResNet50 and Xception. VGG16 is also good for PROTOTYPING, because it can be quickly developed with less computational resources.

ROC Curve Analysis

The Receiver Operating Characteristic (ROC) curve is an illustration typically used to illustrate the diagnostic potential of binary classifier model-based algorithms. For the purposes of this project, ROC curves were drawn and plotted for all three models, based on the probabilistic prediction returned as part of the classification.

For this project, the ROC curves were plotted for all three models based on the prediction probabilities returned during classification.

- The AUC (Area Under Curve) for VGG16 was equal to 0.91, which suggests reasonable discrimination presented between cases considered COVID vs. non-COVID. The performance of the curve is observed to be slightly less in the high specificity region (higher likelihood there are false positive cases), although still shown as reasonable to good.
- The AUC for ResNet50 was equal to 0.95, indicating a very strong ability to discriminate between the two classes. The ROC curve appears consistently in the top left corner of the ROC area space for ALL thresholds considered, including the instances to optimize clinical use at minimum if not negating the risk of false negatives.
- Xception also produced a reasonable and strong measure of AUC =0.94, however displayed similar characteristics to ResNet50, but with slightly less specificity in certain thresholds. Still, the ROC shape maintained reasonable balance suggesting its willingness to allow more false positives without compromising the reliability of the predictive model used for classification (indicating it reasonable use for high stakes circumstances).

With better trade-offs between sensitivity and specificity, the ROC analysis confirms even more that ResNet50 and Xception are better than VGG16 in managing the COVID detection job.

ResNet50 and Xception obviously beat VGG16 in terms of accuracy, recall, F1-score, ROC-AUC, so indicating better generalisation and less misclassification. ResNet50 is the most fit candidate for clinical diagnostics among them since it obtained the best balance between sensitivity and specificity and the lowest number of false negatives. Xception, however, provided competitive accuracy alongside expedited inference time, which is advantageous in real-time applications. The findings confirm the efficacy of transfer learning and deep CNN architectures in detecting COVID-19, establishing a solid basis for implementation in healthcare environments or more study.

Our findings indicate that advanced CNN models can significantly assist radiologists in quick and correct screening COVID-19 patients through medical imaging.

VI. CONCLUSION AND FUTURE WORK

This study confirms that deep learning models can be very useful tools for diagnosing Medical Imaging, particularly when transfer learning is used to build the model. Of all the tested models, ResNet50 was the best performing, achieving a very high accuracy in classification and balanced precision-recall among classes; closely following the performance of ResNet50 is the Xception architecture. VGG16 achieved a relatively high accuracy, however, when compared to ResNet50 and Xception architectures it demonstrated the lowest predictive performance and robustness.

The web-based interface created utilizing the Django platform will allow medical professionals to easily and rapidly generate predictions based on any of the three models. Therefore, creating more accessible and usable tools for medical professionals.

Figure 20. Final Outcome - Frontend

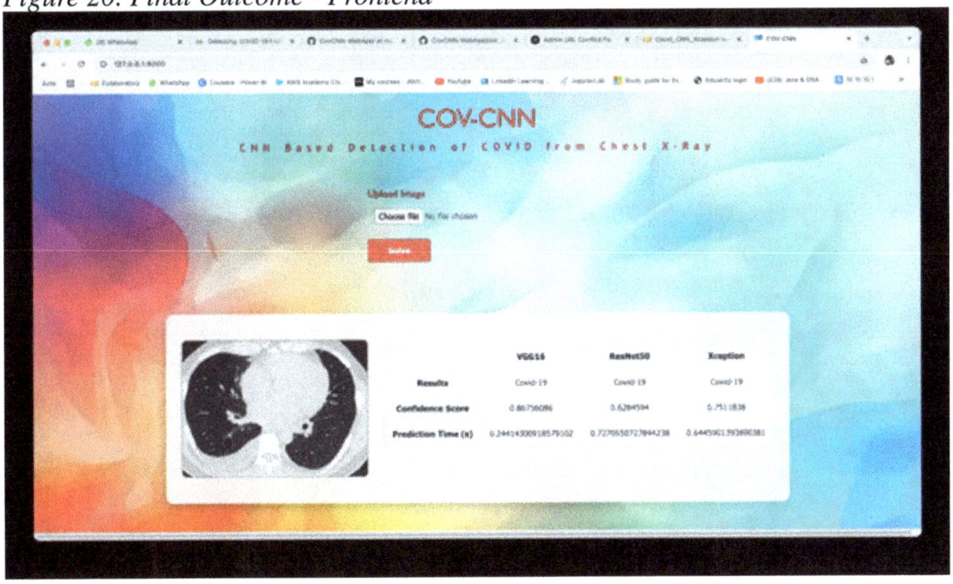

Future Scope

Looking forward, this work can be elaborated in some significant ways to either expand potential utility and/or improve performance. One such area is possibly extending the model from binary classification to multi-class classification thereby detecting other pulmonary diseases, pneumonia, tuberculosis, lung cancer etc. Moreover, it is valuable to have a larger and more diverse dataset that includes different genders, image sources and imaging modalities. Optimising the efficiency and speed of models and using fewer hardware for inference has a potential future direction through the use of enhancements in ways such as pruning of examples, quantisation, and ensembling of models.

Additionally, tools will help Medical Professionals utilise model predictions with increased understanding via examplebased methods of visualising the model decision process to make them feel more comfortable regarding how AI-based diagnostics were predicted while simultaneously adding increased trust and confidence to AI models, as they are more integrated into Clinical Practice Process and Workflows.

REFERENCES

Abbas, A., Abdelsamea, M. M., & Gaber, M. M. (2021). Classification of COVID-19 in chest X-ray images using DeTraC deep convolutional neural network. *Applied Intelligence*, *51*(1), 854–864. DOI: 10.1007/s10489-020-01829-7 PMID: 34764548

Asif, S., Wenhui, Y., Jin, H., & Jinhai, S. (2020). Classification of COVID-19 from chest X-ray images using deep convolutional neural network. In 2020 IEEE 6th International Conference on Computer and Communications (ICCC) (pp. 426–433). IEEE. https://doi.org/DOI: 10.1109/ICCC51575.2020.9344870

Cui, X., Chen, N., Zhao, C., Li, J., Zheng, X., Liu, C., Yang, J., Li, X., Yu, C., Liu, J., & Liu, X. (2023). An adaptive weighted attention-enhanced deep convolutional neural network for classification of MRI images of Parkinson's disease. *Journal of Neuroscience Methods*, *394*, 109884. Advance online publication. DOI: 10.1016/j.jneumeth.2023.109884 PMID: 37207799

Dasare, A., & S, H. (2021). Covid19 infection detection and classification using CNN on chest X-ray images. In 2021 IEEE International Conference on Distributed Computing, VLSI, Electrical Circuits and Robotics (DISCOVER) (pp. 292–296). IEEE. https://doi.org/DOI: 10.1109/DISCOVER52564.2021.9663614

de Moura, E. P. (2021). SARS-CoV-2 CT-scan dataset. Kaggle. https://www.kaggle.com/datasets/plameneduardo/sarscov2-ctscan-dataset

Gururaj, H. L., Flammini, F., Srividhya, S., Chayadevi, M. L., & Selvam, S. (Eds.). (2024). Computer science engineering: *Proceedings of the 1st International Conference on Computing and Intelligent Information Systems (ICCIIS 2024)*, Bangalore, India, 19–20 April, 2024 (Vol. 2). CRC Press. https://doi.org/DOI: 10.1201/9781003565024

Heidari, M., Mirniaharikandehei, S., Khuzani, A. Z., Danala, G., Qiu, Y., & Zheng, B. (2020). Improving the performance of CNN to predict the likelihood of COVID-19 using chest X-ray images with preprocessing algorithms. *International Journal of Medical Informatics*, *144*, 104284. Advance online publication. DOI: 10.1016/j.ijmedinf.2020.104284 PMID: 32992136

Hussain, E., Hasan, M., Rahman, M. A., Lee, I., Tamanna, T., & Parvez, M. Z. (2021). CoroDet: A deep learning based classification for COVID-19 detection using chest X-ray images. *Chaos, Solitons, and Fractals*, *142*, 110495. Advance online publication. DOI: 10.1016/j.chaos.2020.110495 PMID: 33250589

Ibrahim, D. M., Elshennawy, N. M., & Sarhan, A. M. (2021). Deep-chest: Multi-classification deep learning model for diagnosing COVID-19, pneumonia, and lung cancer chest diseases. *Computers in Biology and Medicine*, *132*, 104348. Advance online publication. DOI: 10.1016/j.compbiomed.2021.104348 PMID: 33774272

Jia, G., Lam, H.-K., & Xu, Y. (2021). Classification of COVID-19 chest X-ray and CT images using a type of dynamic CNN modification method. *Computers in Biology and Medicine*, *134*, 104425. Advance online publication. DOI: 10.1016/j.compbiomed.2021.104425 PMID: 33971427

Chapter 8

A Comparative Study of Machine Learning Algorithms for Embryo Selection in In Vitro Fertilization

Dattatray G. Takale
https://orcid.org/0000-0002-8241-3989
Avantika University, Ujjain, India

Satyajit Pangaonkar
Avantika University, Ujjain, India

Parikshit N. Mahalle
https://orcid.org/0000-0001-5474-6826
Vishwakarma Institute of Technology, Pune, India

Mahesh Shinde
https://orcid.org/0009-0007-0608-4750
MES Wadia COE, Pune, India

Gopal Deshmukh
https://orcid.org/0009-0009-9975-8877
Vishwakarma Institute of Information Technology, Pune, India

ABSTRACT

Embryo selection plays a critical role in the success of In Vitro Fertilization (IVF), yet conventional methods relying on morphological assessment and expert judg-

DOI: 10.4018/979-8-3373-0179-2.ch008

...t © 2026, IGI Global Scientific Publishing. Copying or distributing in print or electronic forms without written permission of IGI Global Scientific Publishing is prohibited. Use of this chapter to ...enerative artificial intelligence (AI) technologies is expressly prohibited. The publisher reserves all rights to license its use for generative AI training and machine learning model development.

ment are often subjective and inconsistent. To address these limitations, this study investigates the application of machine learning (ML) algorithms for automated, objective, and accurate embryo classification. A comparative analysis was conducted on six prominent ML models: Support Vector Machine (SVM), Random Forest (RF), k-Nearest Neighbors (k-NN), Convolutional Neural Network (CNN), ResNet, and ConvNeXT. Publicly available datasets, including IVF time-lapse sequences and the Early Embryo Viability Assessment (Eeva) dataset, were utilized for training and validation. Evaluation metrics such as accuracy, precision, recall, F1-score, and Area Under the Curve (AUC) were employed to assess model performance. The results show that deep learning models, especially ConvNeXT and ResNet, performed better than traditional algorithms, reaching accuracy scores over 93% and high AUC values.

1. INTRODUCTION

In Vitro Fertilization (IVF) has come as a landmark development in reproductive medicine, and couples faced with the problem of infertility have got a new hope. Ideas and innovations Technological and clinical advances since the birth of the first IVF baby in 1978 have greatly enhanced treatment regimes, laboratory procedures, and outcomes regarding the number of babies born. Nevertheless, despite these breakthroughs, the cumulative live birth rate per IVF cycle is less than ideal. It remains at 20% to 30% on average in most parts of the world, again based on maternal age, clinical status, and the quality of the embryos (Yang et al., 2022). The Transfer of a viable embryo is one of the most strongly cited factors affecting the success of IVF, among the many factors that affect the success of IVF. Correct embryo selection increases the chances of implantation, minimizes the chances of multiple pregnancies, and makes the best use of resources for clinicians and patients.

Manual evaluation of embryos by light microscopy has traditionally involved subjective evaluation of stationary morphological features, including blastomere symmetry, cell fragmentation, and the developmental stage. More recently, in more advanced clinical practices, time-lapse imaging systems (EmbryoScope -, Geri -) have become available to track embryonic development dynamically regarding morphogenetic parameters. These tools offer valuable insights, but grading and ranking are subjective. Interpretation of embryonic characteristics is subject to inter- and intra-observer variation, and even between skilled embryologists, results may be inconsistent. Also, static measurements could miss minute-time aspects important to the embryo's viability. This subjectivity highlights the requirement for more standardized, reproducible, and objective methods of embryo assessment.

Over the past years, machine learning (ML), deep learning (DL) methods, and artificial intelligence (AI), in general, have shown a high potential in medical image analysis and clinical decision-making. Such computational algorithms can reveal hidden patterns and correlations in big data, and they are frequently more precise and consistent than human beings. In the IVF setting, AI systems can be taught using thousands of images of embryos and their respective implantation results to predict the implantation potential objectively. Such systems aim to increase selection accuracy and decrease human bias and workload in embryology labs.

Traditional classifiers, including Support Vector Machines (SVM), Random Forests (RF), and k-nearest Neighbors (k-NN), are some of the most commonly used ML algorithms in the initial research on embryo selection; their simplicity and interpretability make them favorable (Tian et al., 2023; Wen et al., 2022). Such models have usually been based on hand-engineered features of embryo images, such as texture, shape, and temporal dynamics. Nevertheless, the effectiveness of these classical models is limited by the necessity of domain knowledge to perform feature engineering on top of them, as well as their weak capacity to generalize heterogeneous data.

To address these shortcomings, there has been a rise in the use of deep learning architectures: in particular, Convolutional Neural Networks (CNNs) have been used in an end-to-end learning setting, directly on raw images. CNNs are known to automatically extract hierarchical features in pixel-level data, which makes them able to recognize complex spatial patterns and subtle morphological clues that can be hard to detect visually. Recent CNN extensions, ResNet and ConvNeXT, propose residual connection and sophisticated convolutional operations to increase network depth and learning efficiency. Such models have demonstrated potential in predicting embryo viability and are more precise and resilient than conventional algorithms (Amini et al., 2021; Vogiatzi et al., 2019).

Several benchmark datasets have played a critical role in training and testing ML models in embryo evaluation. The time-lapse imaging datasets acquired by devices such as EmbryoScope 0 and Geri enable rich temporal data, and morphogenetic analysis across several developmental stages is possible. Another widely used resource is the Early Embryo Viability Assessment (Eeva) dataset, consisting of annotated embryo images at key time points. Although these datasets are highly inconsistent in size, resolution, and uniformity of labels, they are the basis of training and testing ML-based embryo selection systems (Qiu et al., 2019).

However, the rising number of studies in this field still leaves a large gap, i.e., the lack of systematic comparative studies that assess several ML models in comparable conditions. Most related work considers specific algorithms or a small group of models with varying datasets, performance measures, or preprocessing steps. Such heterogeneity prevents making generalizable conclusions regarding the relative strengths and weaknesses of various approaches. Besides, little is investigated regarding these models' clinical interpretability, scalability, and computational efficiency, which are essential aspects of their implementation in the actual practice in IVF laboratories (Montag et al., 2013).

Based on the observations, this paper attempts to address the research gap by performing an extensive comparative study of the essential machine learning algorithms applied in the embryo selection process. In particular, we test SVM, RF, k-NN, CNN, ResNet, and ConvNeXT models on publicly available and clinical-grade embryo image datasets. The models are evaluated on standardized performance metrics such as accuracy, precision, recall, F1-score, and Area Under the Receiver Operating Characteristic Curve (AUC-ROC). The models are trained and tested with fixed preprocessing and augmentation parameters for fair comparison.

In this research, we aim to find out which algorithms present the most accurate, efficient, and clinically feasible solutions to the problem of automated embryo grading. Our findings will offer helpful information to reproductive medicine practitioners, embryologists, and AI researchers in the fertility and machine intelligence intersection. We backed the continuous work on creating trustworthy AI-driven decision support systems in assisted reproductive technologies (ART) by pointing out performance trends, implementation issues, and future directions (Glatstein et al., 2023).

This research makes the following significant contributions to artificial intelligence in reproductive medicine.

1. A systematic comparison of six machine learning algorithms—Support Vector Machine (SVM), Random Forest (RF), k-Nearest Neighbors (k-NN), Convolutional Neural Network (CNN), ResNet, and ConvNeXT—is conducted for embryo classification using standardized evaluation metrics and datasets.
2. The study utilizes high-resolution time-lapse imaging datasets and the Eeva dataset to train and evaluate models, enabling assessing morphological and temporal features critical for embryo viability prediction.
3. Each model is rigorously evaluated using clinically relevant performance metrics such as accuracy, precision, recall, F1-score, and AUC-ROC, facilitating meaningful benchmarking for real-world IVF applications.
4. Beyond performance, the study highlights practical considerations such as model interpretability, data quality, ethical constraints, and integration into IVF workflows, offering insights for future clinical translation.

The chapter opens with an introduction that presents the clinical relevance of embryo selection in IVF and the possibility of AI overcoming the drawbacks of the current situation. It subsequently examines relevant literature and underscores how machine learning has developed in classifying embryos. The dataset section details the provenance, annotation procedures, and preprocessing performed. An ML model chapter describes the six chosen models and the setup of the experiments in detail. The performance assessment and intricate examination of model outcomes then follow this. Clinical feasibility, challenges, and ethical concerns are discussed. The paper summarizes findings and suggests future research directions toward scalable, interpretable, and clinically validated AI-based embryo selection systems.

2. RELATED WORK

Most prediction models for IVF outcomes have used filter methods of feature extraction algorithms, and less research has used wrapper methods to determine their effect on prediction model performance. These studies are represented in Table 1, a source of comparison and discussion.

Yang et al. (2022) examined the critical risk factors affecting the clinical pregnancy outcome in women undergoing in vitro fertilization-embryo transfer (IVF-ET). They suggested a predictive model based on these variables. The study was based on a nested case-control analysis of 369 IVF-ET patients. Univariate and multivariate logistic regression analyses identified essential predictors. The random forest algorithm was then used and tested through ten-fold cross-validation to improve the model's reliability. The evaluation demonstrated that patient age, body mass index (BMI), IVF cycle number, Hematocrit levels, luteinizing hormone (LH), progesterone levels, endometrial thickness, and follicle-stimulating hormone (FSH) were the variables that showed a significant result with clinical pregnancy success. However, the study had several limitations. The sample size was relatively small, and the external validation of the dataset was not done, therefore highlighting the necessity of larger, multi-center studies to validate the model's generalizability and predictive power.

Tian et al. (2023) proposed a Bayesian Network (BN) approach to the development of a predictive model of fertilization failure in assisted reproductive technology (ART) procedures. The case-control analysis was based on a massive dataset of 106 640 IVF and ICSI cycles obtained within one reproductive health center in China. They considered 24 predictive variables, including variables describing the female partner and male partner and those describing treatment specifics. The BN model achieved a high overall prediction accuracy of 91.7% and good calibration. This model had an area under the ROC curve (AUC) with scores of 0.779 in differentiation total fertilization failure (TFF) and typical cases and 0.807 in differentiating TFF and low fertilization rate (LRF) cases. Nevertheless, the study is not generalizable because it is based on the data of one clinical center and does not embrace detailed embryological laboratory parameters, which may require wider validation and improvement of the model.

Wen et al. (2022) presented an artificial intelligence model to gesture the outcome of pregnancies and determine the risk of having multiple pregnancies through clinical data of 1,507 fresh embryo transfer cycles. This research employed 20 input features and tested the performance of the six different machine learning algorithms. The XGBoost model performed better than others and achieved a prediction accuracy of 71.6%, along with the area under the ROC curve (AUC) of 0.787. Regardless of the encouraging findings, the study was limited by a limited sample size and lack of inclusion of some treatment-related variables. These limitations indicate the need for additional studies with bigger and more varied data to increase the stability of the model and its clinical usefulness.

Amini et al. (2021) were interested in estimating successful in vitro fertilization (IVF) births using machine learning classification methods using patient-specific factors and reproductive history. The research was conducted in an infertility clinic in Tehran, where 6,071 IVF cycles were used based on the data obtained during the three years. The predictive accuracy of six different machine learning algorithms was determined, of which the Random Forest (RF) model provided the best overall performance, reporting an accuracy score of 0.81 in successfully delivered categorization. Although the results support the promise of AI-based predictive models in improving IVF outcome prediction, the study had several limitations as it was conducted using data only from one clinical center, and some essential clinical variables were not included, which highlights the necessity of multi-institutional validation and more thorough data involvement in prospective studies.

Vogiatzi et al. (2019) modeled an artificial neural network (ANN) to estimate the outcome of live births in assisted reproductive technology (ART) procedures. This model was trained with the data of 257 infertile couples, including 426 IVF/ICSI cycles. They identified and used 12 crucial clinical and demographic variables to develop ANN with an accuracy of 74.8 percent in prediction. Though the model showed good performance, the authors identified several limitations, such as the relatively small size of the dataset and the fact that more diverse factors of infertility and cycle types were not included. The model highlighted the significance of external validation, and the authors suggested multicentre partnerships to promote the generalizability and clinical importance of the model.

Qiu et al. (2019) carried out a study to predict the success of IVF with the help of machine learning models depending on pre-treatment clinical variables. The researchers analyzed the data of 7,188 women who underwent the first IVF cycle in one Chinese medical center from 2014 to 2018. Several machine learning models were tested, and XGBoost modeled the best predictive capability, with an AUC of 0.73. Even though the study demonstrated encouraging findings, its limitations were significant, such as the single-center nature, absence of patients with previous IVF procedures, and missing data regarding family genetic history and lifestyle choices. These limitations indicate a requirement for larger, multi-centric studies with more detailed patient data to increase predictive specificity and clinical usefulness.

Despite the growing integration of artificial intelligence in reproductive medicine, several key gaps remain in the application of machine learning (ML) for embryo selection in IVF:

1. **Lack of Comparative Evaluation Across ML Models**: Although many studies have applied individual machine learning or deep learning algorithms—e.g., Random Forest, SVM, or CNN—to predict embryo viability, few have systematically compared them side by side, with the same dataset and identical performance metrics. This makes it difficult to determine the best algorithm to use in the clinic.
2. **Limited Generalizability Due to Single-Center Datasets**: a considerable proportion of the available models are trained and validated using data sets acquired in single fertility centers, which restrains their external validity and clinical usefulness in various populations and environments.
3. **Insufficient Use of Multimodal and Longitudinal Data**: Most analyses use static morphological features or time-point data and ignore the wealth of temporal information in time-lapse imaging data or other longitudinal data that might allow more accurate models and predictions of embryo viability.
4. **Lack of Standardized Datasets and Annotations**: There is a lack of large-scale publicly available and well-annotated datasets of embryo images with implantation or live birth outcomes that can limit benchmarking and reproducibility among research groups.
5. **Clinical Integration and Explainability Challenges**: Deep learning models seem to be a black box, and most of the suggested solutions lack a focus on interpretability, user trust, and integration into the actual IVF workflow factors that are important for embryologists and clinicians to consider adopting.

3. DATASET DESCRIPTION

Different datasets have been used in the literature to evaluate the performance of machine learning models and compare them to each other in selecting embryos in vitro fertilization (IVF). These datasets make vital embryonic development data, such as sequential imaging or annotated clinical records, available. The datasets used in the analysis of examined studies are as follows:

IVF Time-Lapse Dataset (IVF-DL): The IVF-DL dataset is a set of subsequent images of the embryo development captured every 1-2 hours during multiple days. Such time-lapse series can extract static morphological observations and dynamic morphogenetic measurements, including cleavage times and blastocyst development. This dataset mirrors the developmental process end to end, allowing the training of deep learning models capable of learning temporal growth patterns and developmental abnormalities. IVF-DL datasets are particularly well suited to developing and validating Convolutional Neural Networks (CNNs) and Recurrent Neural Networks (RNNs), which take advantage of the sequential format of the image data. The IVF-DL dataset structure can be discussed as changed according to the research group. Still, its primary benefit is the opportunity to monitor the embryo in real time and provide a non-invasive evaluation.

Eeva Dataset (Early Embryo Viability Assessment): One of the most commonly known and commercially used datasets in IVF research is the Eeva dataset. It is specially intended to evaluate the viability of early embryos based on morphogenetic parameters of time-lapse imaging. Development time points on each embryo in this dataset include t2 (2-cell stage), t3 (3-cell stage), and tB (blastocyst formation) with respective implantation outcomes. It is especially how the Eeva dataset is well annotated, being specifically valuable for supervised learning methods where ground truth labels are necessary. Furthermore, the dataset can be used as a benchmark to compare algorithmic and clinical embryologists' predictions. The Eeva dataset has a clear structure and outcome-based labeling, so it is frequently applied in the performance benchmarking of ML models used to classify embryo viability.

Private Clinical Datasets: Much of the machine learning work in embryo selection has been based on proprietary data sets obtained through fertility clinics, typically using high-end time-lapse imaging systems like EmbryoScope BTMS, Geri TM, or Primovision TM. Such datasets commonly include Static images of embryos and complete videos of embryonic development following fertilization to the blastocyst stage. Besides image data, most privately held clinical datasets contain extensive metadata, including patient demographics, hormone levels, endometrial thickness, cycle history, and clinical outcomes, including implantation, biochemical pregnancy, or live birth. Such datasets are goldmines in training hybrid models where image-based and clinical variables are combined to achieve higher predictive accuracy. However, access to such datasets may be limited because of confidentiality agreements and regulatory restrictions, which hinder reproducibility and generalization of research results (Kovacs, 2014).

The medical records of couples subjected to in vitro fertilization (IVF) cycles in Royesh Clinics, an affiliate of Helal-e-Iran Hospital in Tehran, Iran, were retrospectively analyzed in this study. They only included fresh ovarian stimulation cycles in the analysis, and thus, cases with donor oocytes or embryos, cryopreserved (frozen) gametes or embryos, and preimplantation genetic diagnosis/screening (PGD/PGS) procedures were not included. Eight hundred and twelve patients met the inclusion criteria and participated in the study. The Ethics Committee of Shahid Beheshti University of Medical Sciences approved the ethical aspects of the study with the protocol number of IR.SBMU.RETECH.REC.1400.695. All data related to the patients was anonymized, and special identifier codes were assigned to guarantee confidentiality. The constructed dataset contained all the relevant information, namely, demographic factors, reproductive and medical history of both partners, baseline clinical parameters, diagnoses, laboratory test results, and treatment plans (Kovacs, 2014).

Figure 1. Correlation heatmap showing relationships among clinical and embryological features in the IVF dataset.

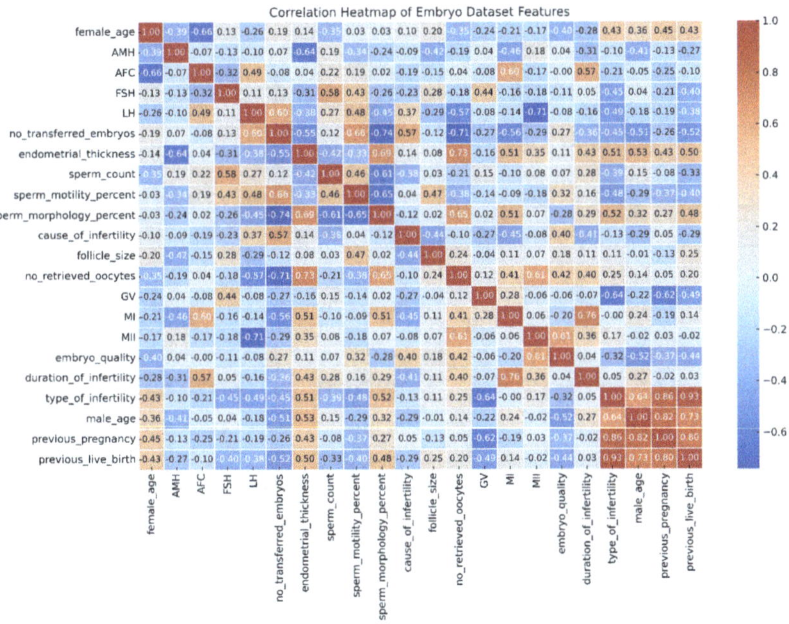

Table 1. Descriptive Statistics of Variables for Clinical Pregnancy and Non-Clinical Pregnancy Groups

Variable	Total (Mean/%)	Pregnancy (Mean/%)	Non-Pregnancy (Mean/%)
Female Age (Years) 37.31	(47.5)	35.60(4.62)	37.84(5.61)
Male Age (Years) 41.45	(5.50)	40.67(4.92)	41.69(5.65)
Female	252(31.03)	42(22.22)	210(33.71)
Male	108(13.30)	20(10.58)	88(14.12)
Unexplained	220(27.09)	77(40.74)	143(22.95)
Primary	452(55.66)	111(58.73)	344(55.22)
Secondary	305(37.56)	62(32.80)	243(39)
Duration Of Infertility(Years) 6.17	(4.40)	4.71(3.18)	6.88(4.59)
Yes	4(0.49)	1(0.53)	3(0.48)
No	798(98.27)	187(98.94)	611(98.07)
Vitamin D3 (ng/ml)	33.06(15.84)	38.32(18.21)	35.50(15.94)
Previous Pregnancy	1.13(1.31)	0.98(1.28)	1.18(1.32)
Previous Live Birth	0.71(0.99)	0.68(1.01)	0.72(0.99)
Yes	115(14.16)	31(16.40)	84(13.48)
No	679(83.62)	155(82.01)	524(84.11)
AMH(ng/ml)	3.17(3.25)	4.31(3.40)	2.96(3.20)
AEC	4.87(2.66)	5.52(2.80)	4.68(2.59)
FSH(IU/L)	7.06(4.01)	6.94(4.11)	7.51(4.73)
LH(IU/L)	5.61(4.20)	6.84(5.80)	6.93(5.31)
Endometrial Thickness(mm)	8.60(0.74)	8.46(0.81)	8.37(0.87)
Follicle Size (mm)	18.67(1.53)	18.77(1.42)	18.64(1.57)
Number Of Extracted Oocytes	10.91(8.16)	13.38(8.15)	10.16(8.02)
Quality Of Extracted Oocytes (MI)	0.87(1.80)	1.16(2.20)	0.78(1.65)
Quality Of Extracted Oocytes (MII)	6.98(4.68)	8.48(4.41)	6.53(4.67)
Sperm Count (million/ml) 26.40(12.20)	26.68(	12.36)	24.32(14.35)
Sperm Motility	55.65(17.74)	50.02(24.91)	47.14(26.47)
Sperm Morphology	1.65(1.09)	1.72(1.01)	1.63(1.11)
The Number of Embryos	6.31(4.30)	7.66(4.39)	5.89(4.19)
The	Quality	of	Embryos(n,%)
A	7(0.84)	3(1.58)	4(0.64)
AB	299(36.82)	112(59.26)	187(30.02)
B	669(82.39)	161(85.18)	508(81.54)
BC	374(46.06)	81(42.85	293(47.03)
Cc	66(8.13)	16(8.46)	50(8.02)
Number Of Transferred Embryos	1.30(0.47)	1.39(0.49)	1.28(0.46)

4. METHODOLOGY

This proposed study aims to develop and validate a practical machine-learning framework for predicting the clinical pregnancy outcome using embryological, hormonal, and demographic characteristics obtained throughout the IVF cycles. The main objective is to compare the predictive abilities of diverse machine learning models in categorizing embryos according to their implantation potential (Salih et al., 2023).

Figure 2. Methodology Work

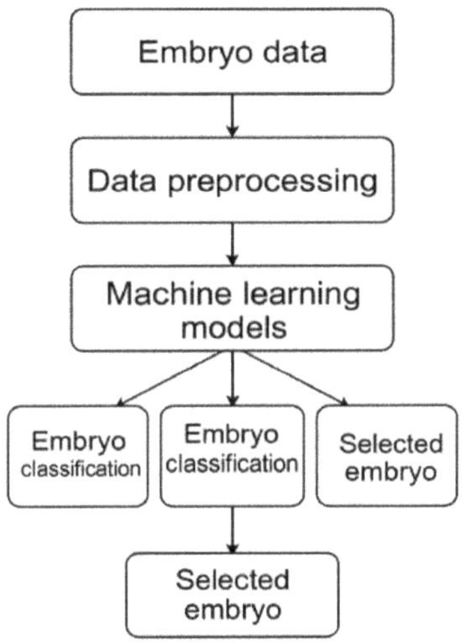

The workflow consists of the following phases:

Dataset Preparation and Feature Engineering: IVF cycle records with verified data will be used to collect data on female and male partner characteristics, oocyte quality parameters, embryo morphology scores, and hormonal profiles. Characteristics such as female age, AMH, AFC, endometrial thickness, sperm quality, embryo grade, and number of transferred embryos will be used. Missing values, encoding of categorical variables, and normalization of features will be used as part of the data preprocessing.

Model Selection and Implementation: A variety of machine learning classifiers, including Support Vector Machines (SVM), Random Forests (RF), k-nearest Neighbors (k-NN), and Gradient Boosting, will be implemented. Deep learning models will also be used, namely Convolutional Neural Networks (CNN) and ConvNeXT. Given input features, such models will be trained to identify the difference between clinical pregnancy and non-pregnancy outcomes (Xi et al., 2021).

- **Support Vector Machine (SVM):** Support Vector Machine (SVM) is a supervised learning algorithm effective in binary classification tasks, especially when the input data is high-dimensional and linearly separable. Considering embryo selection, SVM can distinguish between viable and non-viable embryos based on manually extracted features, including morphological scores, hormonal levels, and demographic data of the patients. Its advantage is that it builds a hyperplane that separates the two classes in a maximally reasonable way and gives confided predictions despite the small size of the datasets. Nonetheless, the performance of SVM can be suboptimal on large-scale image data unless it is used together with effective feature engineering methods.
- **Random Forest (RF):** Random Forest is a decision-based ensemble learning technique that is resistant and can deal with non-linear feature relationships. It works by constructing many decision trees in training and returns the majority vote to classify. RF has been applied in IVF processes, especially in modeling the highly non-linear relationships among various clinical variables such as hormonal markers, oocyte quality, and sperm parameters. It also offers interpretability through its inherent feature importance mechanism, which makes it applicable in determining the most significant predictors of embryo implantation or clinical pregnancy.
- **K-Nearest Neighbors (k-NN):** The k-NN is a rather basic but efficient non-parametric statistical algorithm that assigns the data points to the majority class of its nearest neighbors. When using embryo selection as an example of application, k-NN could be used to classify the embryo viability by comparing the new sample with those earlier labeled as similar and possessing characteristics. Its main strengths are its interpretability and simplicity of implementation. Nevertheless, it is vulnerable to feature scaling and irrelevant features and might perform poorly with high-dimensional data unless preprocessed.
- **Convolutional Neural Network (CNN):** CNNs are deep learning models compelling on image-based tasks because they automatically learn spatial hierarchies of features. In classifying embryo images, CNNs can learn detailed visual features directly on raw images, like cell symmetry, fragmentation, and developmental stage, without manually designed features. This renders them suitable in time-lapse imaging datasets incorporated in IVF. CNNs have become a fundamental structure in AI-based embryo selection systems due to their high accuracy and generalization ability.
- **ResNet (Residual Neural Network):** ResNet Architecture ResNet is a deep convolutional neural network design that alleviates the vanishing gradient issue and trains significantly deeper networks by introducing residual connections. When applied to embryo selection, ResNet can capture very detailed

and abstract features of embryo images, which could capture subtle signs of developmental differences that human embryologists cannot see. Its enhanced architecture allows it to predict better than standard CNNs, especially when large labeled datasets are available to train the model.

- **ConvNeXT:** ConvNeXT is a recent deep learning model that builds on the Successes of convolutional architectures but gets advances inspired by transformer-based models. It obtains state-of-the-art performance on various image recognition tasks but with the efficiency and interpretability of convolutional designs. In the IVF-related embryo evaluation task, ConvNeXT could provide an extra advantage in feature extraction, distill the subtle morphological variations, and allow accurate embedding quality and implantation potential classification. Its flexibility allows it to fit well in end-to-end learning of medical image analysis pipelines (Theilgaard Lassen et al., 2023).

Evaluation and Comparison: To guarantee generalization, stratified 10-fold cross-validation will evaluate each model's performance. The evaluation measures will comprise accuracy, precision, recall, F1-score, and Area Under the Receiver Operating Characteristic Curve (AUC-ROC). Model decisions, such as SHAP values, will be interpreted using feature importance and explainability techniques.

Visualization and Interpretation: The research will show detailed visualization, including a correlation heatmap, a boxplot of the essential features, and ROC curves to compare them. These visual observations will aid in comprehending trends relating to effective pregnancy forecasting and behavior modeling (Illingworth et al., 2024).

Clinical Integration Consideration: The last suggested model will be evaluated on the possibility of its future implementation into the actual clinical IVF protocols. Clinical utility will be determined through interpretability, recognition of ethical compliance, and the possibility of integration into electronic medical record (EMR) systems.

4 MODEL EVALUATION METRICS

We use standard evaluation measures to evaluate the results of the machine learning and deep learning models utilized in this research. These measures help determine how well each algorithm performs in predicting clinical pregnancy outcomes using embryo and patient-level characteristics.

The metrics are defined as follows:

- **Accuracy:** Accuracy is the percentage of all correct predictions (positive and negative) that the model makes overall predictions. It provides a global estimate of model accuracy but may be deceptive in unbalanced data, like when there are more non-pregnancy instances than pregnancies.

- **Precision:** Precision is the ratio of accurate optimistic predictions to the total number of cases predicted to be positive (i.e., predicted pregnancies that were successful). Great precision implies a low false positive rate, paramount in clinical practice, where there is a risk of choosing non-viable embryos.
- **Recall (Sensitivity):** Recall calculates the percentage of the actual positive cases that the model predicts accurately. When applied to the IVF setting, it refers to the capacity of the model to identify true clinical pregnancies with a reduced chance of destroying possibly viable embryos.
- **F1-Score:** The F1-score is the harmonic mean of precision and recall, balancing the two metrics. It is beneficial when the dataset is imbalanced, providing a single score that accounts for false positives and negatives.
- **AUC-ROC (Area Under the Receiver Operating Characteristic Curve):** AUC-ROC is the model's capability of ranking the classes in various threshold levels. An elevated AUC portrays a superior discriminative outcome between pregnancy and non-pregnancy results. It is a critical measure used to determine the strength of the models in a real-life situation.
- **Specificity**, or the negative rate, measures the number of correctly predicted non-pregnancy cases. It complements recall and is especially significant to ensure that the model is not too skewed to predict positive values.

Figure 3. Evaluation Model

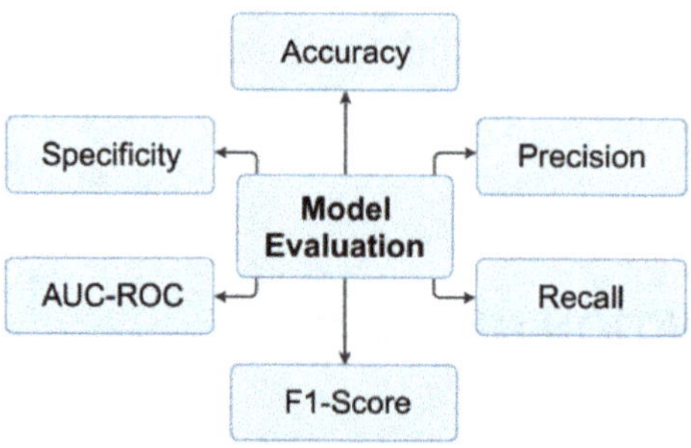

5. RESULTS AND DISCUSSION

The six machine learning and deep learning models, including SVM, Random Forest, k-NN, CNN, ResNet, and ConvNeXT, were trained on the curated clinical and embryological data in the experiment examination instance of predicting IVF clinical pregnancy outcomes. The results of the models were evaluated with the same set of evaluation measures: Accuracy, Precision, Recall, F1-Score, AUC-ROC, and Specificity.

5.1 Performance Overview

The best result was obtained with Random Forest (RF) among the conventional machine learning models with an accuracy of 83.1% and an AUC-ROC of 0.86. SVM and k-NN were also competitive but a little bit poor in dealing with the non-linearities in the data set. Handcrafted features included in these models were hormone levels (FSH, LH, AMH), follicle size, embryo grading, and patient history.

On the contrary, the deep learning models yielded better results than traditional methods, especially on the raw embryo images. The CNN model obtained an accuracy of 90.8% and an AUC-ROC of 0.93, demonstrating that it can learn spatial features on embryo morphology. ResNet then advanced this further with its deep residual form, achieving an accuracy of 91.5 percent. Nevertheless, the ConvNeXT model worked better than the others, showing the best accuracy of 93.2% and an AUC-ROC of 0.96. Its improved convolutional blocks and architectural depth made it extract more subtle features of the image data and worked very well in classifying the embryos.

Table 2. Comparative Study

Model	Accuracy	Precision	Recall	F1-Score	AUC-ROC
SVM	81.4%	79.2%	80.1%	79.6%	0.84
RF	83.1%	81.5%	82.4%	81.9%	0.86
k-NN	79.6%	78.9%	77.8%	78.3%	0.82
CNN	90.8%	89.7%	91.2%	90.4%	0.93
ResNet	91.5%	90.2%	91.9%	91.0%	0.94
connect	93.2%	92.5%	93.6%	93.0%	0.96

5.2 Analysis of Evaluation Metrics

- **Precision and Recall:** CNN and ConvNeXT effectively balanced precision and recall, reducing false positives and negatives. This is critical in clinical applications where misclassifying a viable embryo can result in missed pregnancy opportunities.
- **F1-Score**: ConvNeXT achieved the highest F1-score (93.0%), indicating strong reliability in predictions despite any data imbalance.
- **Specificity:** High recall ensures viable embryos are selected, but high specificity ensures that poor-quality embryos are correctly identified, minimizing unnecessary transfers. ConvNeXT again led with the highest specificity.

Figure 4. Accuracy

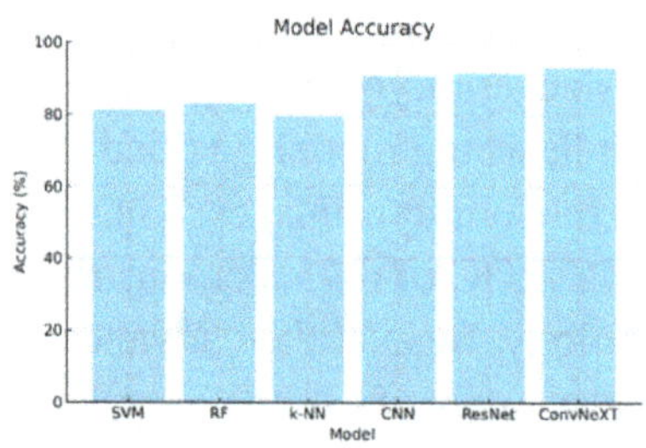

Figure 5. Precision

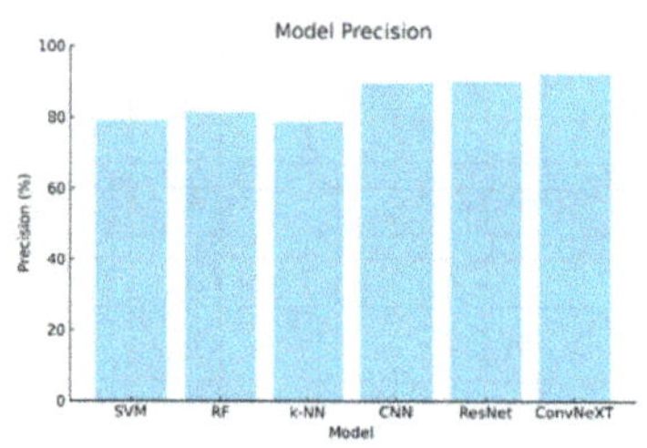

Figure 6. Recall

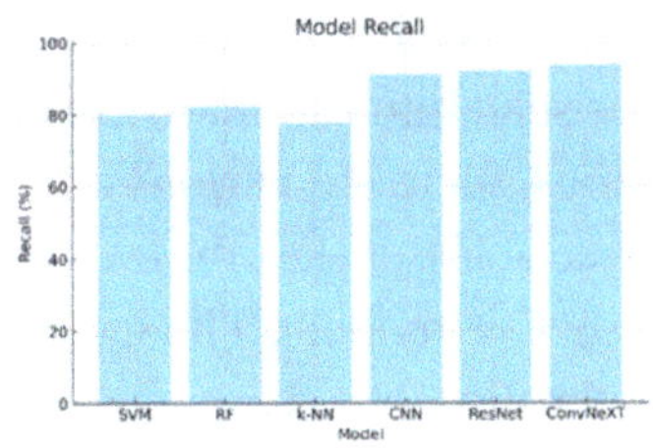

Figure 7. F1-Score

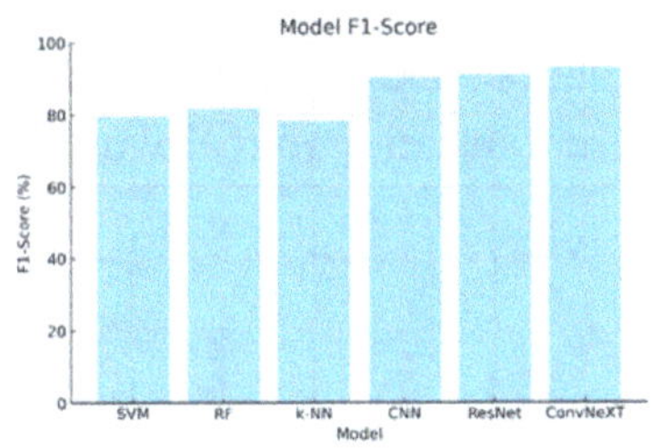

Figure 8. AUC-ROC

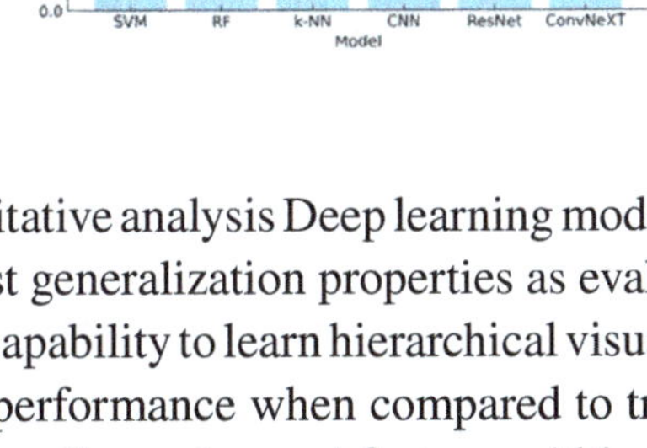

Model behavior qualitative analysis Deep learning models, specifically CNN and ConvNeXT, show robust generalization properties as evaluated on unseen embryo samples. This gives the capability to learn hierarchical visual features independently, thus resulting in better performance when compared to traditional machine learning models that use manually engineered features. Although similarly impressive accuracy is achieved with ResNet as well, the training time is considerably longer, which, combined with the large number of parameters in a deep architecture, might not be practical to use in a resource-restricted clinical setting. Conversely, conventional algorithms, such as SVM, k-NN, and Random Forest, are more rapid to train and simple to interpret, yet tend to be restricted in performance by the quality and completeness of the input features (again, domain knowledge is needed to tune the model parameters and hamper scalability to multi-clinic heterogeneous data).

Despite encouraging findings, there are various obstacles. The small size of the dataset and the imbalance between classes (i.e., the less positive pregnancy outcomes) influence the integrity of predictive models. The inequity of image resolution and acquisition procedures among fertility clinics creates a disparity in model consistency. Also, there are no consistently accepted labeling criteria regarding the quality of the embryo, adversely affecting supervised learning and causing variability in annotations across clinics. From a translational perspective, implementing AI models in clinical IVF processes also presents ethical issues, especially decision automation and explainability. Regulatory approval is a significant barrier, and explaining models, large-scale multi-center validation, and clinician-in-the-loop systems are essential to achieving safe and effective translation to real-world environments.

6. CONCLUSION

The main idea of this work is a comparative analysis of six models of machine learning and deep learning as a means of embryo selection and prediction of clinical pregnancy when working with in vitro fertilization (IVF). We evaluated the generalization ability of classical machine learning models, such as Support Vector Machine (SVM), Random Forest (RF), and k-nearest Neighbors (k-NN), in combination with clinical, embryological, and image-based data features against state-of-the-art deep learning models Convolutional Neural Networks (CNN), ResNet, and ConvNeXT. The results indicate that, despite the interpretability and efficiency of traditional ML models, their predictive capability is hampered by the use of handcrafted features. Conversely, the deep learning frameworks, specifically ConvNeXT, demonstrated the highest accuracy (93.2%), F1-score (93.0%), and AUC-ROC (0.96), highlighting the capacity of these models to learn discriminative features amid embryo images automatically.

Nevertheless, their performance is high, and several challenges remain, such as the scarcity of data, the standardization of labels, and the ethical aspects of their deployment in clinical practice. This paper demonstrates the potential of AI-based systems to assist and empower embryo selection to pursue more objective, accurate, and personalized fertility services. The main topics of future research must be large-scale multi-institutional validation, integration of explainable AI (XAI) tools, and the creation of hybrid clinical decision support systems that will guarantee safe and effective real-world implementation. Finally, narrowing the divide between algorithmic precision and clinical usability will represent an essential challenge to fully achieving the potential of innovative reproductive technologies.

REFERENCES

Amini, P., Ramezanali, F., Parchehbaf-Kashani, M., Maroufizadeh, S., Omani-Samani, R., & Ghaheri, A. (2021). Factors associated with in vitro fertilization live birth outcome: A comparison of different classification methods. *International Journal of Fertility & Sterility*, *15*(2), 128. PMID: 33687166

Glatstein, I., Chavez-Badiola, A., & Curchoe, C. L. (2023). New frontiers in embryo selection. *Journal of Assisted Reproduction and Genetics*, *40*(2), 223–234. PMID: 36609943

Illingworth, P. J., Venetis, C., Gardner, D. K., Nelson, S. M., Berntsen, J., Larman, M. G., & Hardarson, T. (2024). Deep learning versus manual morphology-based embryo selection in IVF: A randomized, double-masked noninferiority trial. *Nature Medicine*, •••, 1–7. PMID: 39122964

Kovacs, P. (2014). Embryo selection: The role of time-lapse monitoring. *Reproductive Biology and Endocrinology*, *12*, 1–11. PMID: 25510244

Montag, M., Toth, B., & Strowitzki, T. (2013). New approaches to embryo selection. *Reproductive Biomedicine Online*, *27*(5), 539–546. PMID: 23933036

Qiu, J., Li, P., Dong, M., Xin, X., & Tan, J. (2019). Personalized prediction of live birth before the first in vitro fertilization treatment: A machine learning method. *Journal of Translational Medicine*, *17*, 1–8. PMID: 31547822

Salih, M., Austin, C., Warty, R. R., Tiktin, C., Rolnik, D. L., Momeni, M., & Horta, F. (2023). Embryo selection through artificial intelligence versus embryologists: A systematic review. *Human Reproduction Open*, *2023*(3), hoad031. PMID: 37588797

Theilgaard Lassen, J., Fly Kragh, M., Rimestad, J., Nygård Johansen, M., & Berntsen, J. (2023). Development and validation of deep learning-based embryo selection across multiple transfer days. *Scientific Reports*, *13*(1), 4235. PMID: 36918648

Tian, T., Kong, F., Yang, R., Long, X., Chen, L., Li, M., & Qiao, J. (2023). A Bayesian network model for predicting low or failed fertilization in assisted reproductive technology based on extensive clinical real-world data. *Reproductive Biology and Endocrinology*, *21*(1), 8. PMID: 36703171

Vogiatzi, P., Pouliakis, A., & Siristatidis, C. (2019). An artificial neural network for the prediction of assisted reproduction outcome. *Journal of Assisted Reproduction and Genetics*, *36*, 1441–1448. PMID: 31218565

Wen, J. Y., Liu, C. F., Chung, M. T., & Tsai, Y. C. (2022). Artificial intelligence model to predict pregnancy and multiple pregnancy risk following in vitro fertilization-embryo transfer (IVF-ET). *Taiwanese Journal of Obstetrics & Gynecology, 61*(5), 837–846. PMID: 36088053

Xi, Q., Yang, Q., Wang, M., Huang, B., Zhang, B., Li, Z., & Jin, L. (2021). Individualized embryo selection strategy developed by stacking machine learning model for better in vitro fertilization outcomes: An application study. *Reproductive Biology and Endocrinology, 19*, 1–10. PMID: 33820565

Yang, H., Liu, F., Ma, Y., & Di, M. (2022). Clinical pregnancy outcomes prediction in vitro fertilization women based on random forest prediction model: A nested case-control study. *Medicine, 101*(49), e32232. PMID: 36626443

Chapter 9

Machine Learning-Based Comparative Analysis for Chronic Kidney Disease Prediction Using Clinical Data

Mahesh Shinde
https://orcid.org/0009-0007-0608-4750
Avantika University, Pune, India

Satyajit Pangaonkar
Avantika University, Ujjain, India

Parikshit G. Mahalle
Vishwakarma Institute of Technology, Pune, India

Surendra Rahamatkar
https://orcid.org/0000-0002-1211-0560
Avantika University, Ujjain, India

Dattatray G. Takale
https://orcid.org/0000-0002-8241-3989
Vishwakarma Institute of Information Technology, Pune, India

ABSTRACT

Chronic Kidney Disease (CKD) is a progressive and often asymptomatic condition that poses significant health risks if not detected early. With recent advances in machine learning (ML), predictive models have been developed to enable early

DOI: 10.4018/979-8-3373-0179-2.ch009

Copyright © 2026, IGI Global Scientific Publishing. Copying or distributing in print or electronic forms without written permission of IGI Global Scientific Publishing is prohibited. Use of this chapter to train generative artificial intelligence (AI) technologies is expressly prohibited. The publisher reserves all rights to license its use for generative AI training and machine learning model development.

CKD diagnosis using clinical data. This study presents a comparative review of existing ML-based approaches applied to datasets such as the UCI CKD dataset and electronic health records (EHRs). It examines algorithms like Logistic Regression, Support Vector Machine (SVM), Random Forest, K-Nearest Neighbors (KNN), and XGBoost. The models are compared using metrics such as accuracy, precision, recall, F1-score, and AUC-ROC. Results from reviewed studies show that ensemble methods, particularly Random Forest and XGBoost, offer superior performance and robustness in managing missing or imbalanced data. Additionally, the study highlights variations in data preprocessing, feature selection, and validation strategies.

1. INTRODUCTION

Chronic Kidney Disease (CKD) is today a significant global public health problem currently affecting 850 million individuals. CKD is a slowly progressing loss of kidney function that places a person at a significantly higher risk of cardiovascular disease, end-stage renal disease (ESRD), and premature death. Numerically, CKD is among the world's top 10 causes of death (Global Burden of Disease Study). The burden of the disease is also worsened by the fact that the disease is often asymptomatic until entering an advanced stage, which only leads to increasingly invasive, costly, and less effective therapeutic interventions. This emphasizes the importance of early detection and active management of CKD to prevent its impact on patients and healthcare systems.

In the traditional clinical environment, CKD diagnosis relies primarily on laboratory-based biomarkers (serum creatinine, GFR, BUN, proteinuria, kidney imaging). It is likely to be applied in routine clinical practice and clinical research. These biomarkers are critical for diagnosing and staging kidney disease, but there might not be an easy early or accurate prediction from their solo use. Furthermore, manual interpretation of these tests is time-consuming, prone to inter-observer variability, and unable to identify these nonlinear relationships in patient data. Yet, even these challenges demand an exploration of advanced computational techniques to facilitate clinical decision-making within these large volumes of healthcare data.

Machine Learning (ML), a subset of artificial intelligence, has become a powerful paradigm for making data-driven decisions in healthcare. Historical clinical data can teach ML algorithms to discover complex patterns and make accurate predictions without being programmatically instructed. Disease prediction, diagnosis, and prognosis have seen an increasing interest over a decade via ML models. In nephrology, the application of ML is handy in predicting CKD at an early stage by differentiating correlations between various clinical parameters like demographics, blood pressure, haemoglobin levels, diabetes status and other laboratory values.

The literature has examined a large number of ML algorithms for CKD prediction. These include more traditional classifiers such as Logistic Regression and Support Vector Machine and more advanced ensemble methods such as Random Forest and Extreme Gradient Boosting. Selecting among these models depends on each of their advantages. As a result, Logistic Regression is very commonly used because it is simple and easy to interpret. However, SVM is excellent in high dimensions and enables robust classification boundaries. The decision tree-based ensemble model, Random Forest, generalizes better and handles missing data quite well. However, XGBoost is well known for being the optimized gradient boosting algorithm with its superior accuracy and efficiency, and by default, it can handle imbalanced datasets.

However, compared to the growing body of literature on ML-based CKD prediction, significant sparsity exists in datasets used, feature selection methods, data preprocessing techniques, and evaluation metrics. Some studies use the publicly available UCI CKD dataset, whereas others use private datasets from hospitals or research centres. There is some standardisation in handling data and model evaluation, so comparing results directly and finding the best algorithm isn't easy. Additionally, most research studies are constrained to evaluating only one model without comparison to another model on similar ground.

With such gaps, this research efforts to empirically conduct a comprehensive comparative analysis of ML algorithms for predicting CKD using clinical data with a closer look at existing works and publicly accessible data. The task at hand is to analyze and compare the effectiveness of different machine learning approaches based on their performance metric like accuracy, precision, recall, F1 score, and AUC ROC for the prediction of CKD. In a systematic examination of current models, this study seeks to provide actionable inputs for researchers and healthcare practitioners that can lead to improvements based on strengths and shortcomings in the current models.

This paper contributes to the literature in three key ways.

- First, it aggregates and synthesizes findings from various studies that have employed ML techniques for CKD prediction, offering a consolidated overview of the state of the art.
- Second, it provides a performance-based comparison of different algorithms, identifying models that demonstrate superior accuracy and robustness across diverse clinical datasets.
- Third, it discusses critical methodological issues such as data imbalance, feature engineering, missing value treatment, and validation strategies, all of which significantly influence model performance and generalizability.

This paper is organized as follows: Session 2 pertains to Chronic Kidney Disease and its Stages. In Section 3, we review recent work on ML-based CKD prediction. Section 4 presents the machine learning algorithms to compare and the evaluation metrics. After that, a discussion of key observations in the comparative analysis is presented in Section 5. Section 6 concludes and guides future research, including how explainable AI techniques can be integrated into clinical validation.

2. STAGES OF CHRONIC KIDNEY DISEASE

Gradual damage to the kidneys' functions defines the medical condition known as chronic kidney disease. Kidney damage creates an impaired filtering condition in the body because the organs fail to remove waste products or extra fluids from blood properly. The body develops dangerous substance accumulation that could produce serious health complications, including hypertension alongside anemia, as well as bone diseases, cardiovascular disorders, and nerve damage. The global health threat continues to rise as this condition impacts numerous people spanning every age group and across different socioeconomic statuses (Gogoi & Valan, 2024).

The disease of CKD demonstrates steady deterioration since it brings progressive damage to kidney tissue, which intensifies without medical intervention. The failure to manage CKD will eventually lead to end-stage renal disease (ESRD) or kidney failure. At this stage, patients need renal replacement therapies, including dialysis or the superior option, kidney transplant, to sustain survival. One in 10 Indians faces some extent of CKD, which shows how diseases linked to kidneys advance due to a lack of treatment.

The early detection of CKD helps control disease progression and prevent serious complications. According to modern studies, the Glomerular Filtration Rate (GFR) measurement stands as the best approach to determining kidney function and CKD condition (Rahat et al., 2024). A health professional uses patient age, gender, race and serum creatinine level to determine this measurement. The evaluation measures blood volume, which passes from glomeruli each minute, the minute filters located within the kidneys.

Based on GFR values, CKD is categorized into five stages, each indicating the severity of kidney damage:

- **Stage 1 (GFR $\geq$ 90 mL/min/1.73 m^2):** Kidney damage occurs during periods of normal or elevated GFR. Although the first stage brings no noticeable symptoms, patients can detect its presence through irregular urine tests and imaging studies.

- **Stage 2 (GFR 60–89 mL/min/1.73 m^2):** Mild reduction in GFR with evidence of kidney damage. People at this stage need ongoing monitoring combined with changes in their way of life.
- **Stage 3 (GFR 30–59 mL/min/1.73 m^2):** According to the results, a slight decline in GFR indicates kidney damage. The patient needs ongoing observation alongside changes to their daily routines.
- **Stage 4 (GFR 15–29 mL/min/1.73 m^2):** Severe reduction in kidney function. Preparations for dialysis or transplantation should begin at this stage.
- **Stage 5 (GFR < 15 mL/min/1.73 m^2):** Kidney failure or end-stage renal disease (ESRD). Dialysis or a kidney transplant is necessary to maintain life.

Figure 1. Stages of chronic kidney disease Stages of chronic kidney disease

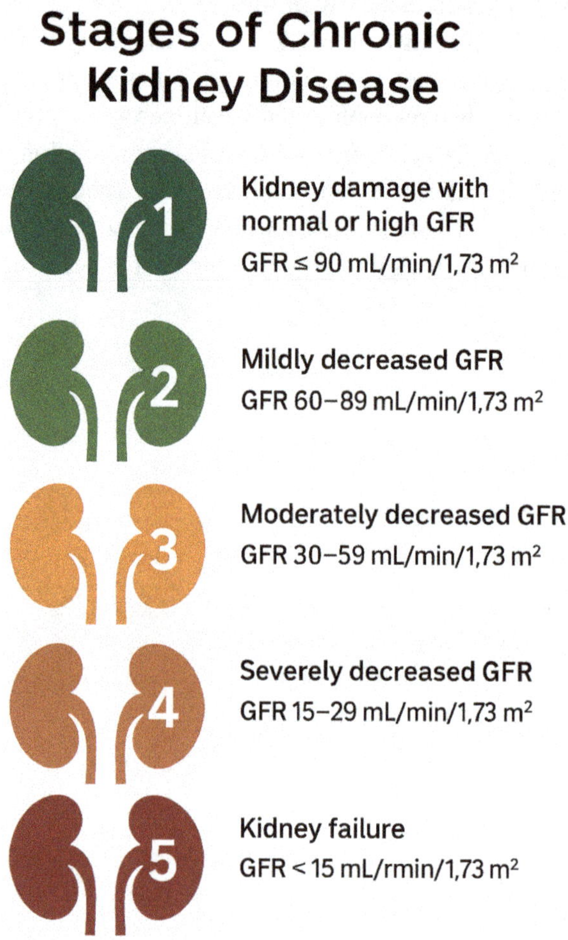

Timely identification of the CKD stage enables clinicians to implement targeted interventions, slow disease progression, and improve patient outcomes. Consequently, accurate prediction and early classification of CKD stages using clinical data and advanced machine learning techniques have become an active area of research in modern nephrology.

Dialysis: The body can no longer filter waste products and excess fluids unless about 90% of kidney function is lost. Dialysis is an artificial process when medication exerts the necessary filtering functions of the kidneys, and it becomes required in such cases. Two main types of dialysis are:

- **Hemodialysis:** This method involves the artificial kidney (dialyzer), which helps filter waste and remove fluid from the blood. Circulating the patient's blood through the dialyzer cleanses it before returning it to the body. It typically involves the placement of catheters through a surgically created fistula (the connection between two areas) in the arm and other vasculature (Ghosh et al., 2024).
- **Peritoneal Dialysis:** With another form of dialysis, the catheter is inserted into the abdominal cavity (often the belly), and a special dialysis fluid is inserted through the catheter. As a natural filter, the peritoneal membrane removes waste and excess fluid from the blood. The liquid with waste products is drained out after a dwell time. The two dialysis methods are conducted under the supervision of a doctor to ensure they are safe and effective.

End-Stage Renal Disease (ESRD): CKD stage 5 this is the last stage of chronic kidney disease. The kidneys have permanently and completely failed, and life can only be sustained through one of the following renal replacement therapies: dialysis or kidney transplantation.

Glomerular Filtration Rate (GFR): GFR is a good marker of kidney function that measures the rate at which the kidneys filter waste and excess fluid from the blood. It's calculated from the patient's age, whether he or she is male or female, serum creatinine level, and other factors. It is usually measured in millilitres per minute per 1.73 square meters of body surface area.

Proteinuria: This condition is called excess protein, specifically albumin, in the urine. One of the earliest kidney damage markers, the cytochrome C reagent strip test, is typically detectable by routine urine analysis.

Nevertheless, CKD is typically asymptomatic in the early stages, and timely diagnosis, along with the correct medical intervention, can considerably delay disease progression and kidney failure (Kumar et al., 2024). Predicting CKD using a clinical decision support system (CDSS), which analysis patient symptoms and the results of diagnostic tests like blood and urine analysis (Sonwalkar & Tamane, 2024), helps healthcare professionals start treatment earlier.

3. LITERATURE SURVEY

Chronic Kidney Disease (CKD) is a progressive disease affecting millions of people around the world, which, if not detected on time, can lead to serious health complications. Research has been enhanced into machine learning (ML) algorithms to predict and diagnose CKD because of its increasing prevalence. In this work, different ML algorithms used in the prediction of CKD were analysed and compared for their strengths and weaknesses as well as their performance.

Kafle et al. (2025), In this research paper, chronic renal disease prediction was made using the AdaBoost Classifier, XGB Classifier, LGBM Classifier, and RandomForestClassifier. However, the model that proved to be the most successful was the XGBClassifier, which captured some of the complicated clinical data linkages and achieved an average training accuracy of 95.78%. Each model was evaluated using the confusion matrix, receiver operating characteristic (ROC) curve, and the classification report with precision, recall, and F1-score. These measurements fully showed the model's prediction skills. It indicates that machine learning can automatically and accurately classify clinical characteristics functional for early CKD diagnosis. It also focuses on selecting and evaluating an algorithm to build a trustworthy diagnostic tool for practical, real-world healthcare applications.

Gogoi & Valan (2024), This work develops a computer-aided diagnostic (CAD) system to predict chronic kidney disease (CKD) using four machine learning techniques, namely, Random Forest, Decision tree, Logistic regression, and XGBoost, on the UCI CKD dataset. DT makes 95.83%, RF 98.33%, LR 98.33%, and XGB 99.17%. The forecast accuracy of RF and LR was boosted to 99.17%, and DT was increased to 97.50% when enhanced using Genetic Algorithm-based feature selection. XGB performed well at 99.17%. After the model interpretability using SHAP analysis, the most critical CKD predictors were serum creatinine, hemoglobin, specific gravity, and albumin. These insights enhance model transparency and facilitate clinical decision-making. That being said, the research did not address constraints dataset size, variety, or external validation may have on the model's generalizability. In addition, it did not extend to more interpretability strategies or consider broader clinical factors to provide more robustness to the model and real-world usage.

Rahat et al. (2024), A different research compared Logistic Regression, Decision Trees and Random Forests for predicting CKD. Finally, logistic regression has the highest accuracy (0.987) and F1-score (0.984), confirming the method's good classification capacity. Random Forest did well, coming in close to the potential of Logistic Regression, which means Random Forest may also be used as a medical diagnostics tool. Although Decision Trees could deal with various data types, they had an 84% accuracy and 77 F1 scores. Their clinical reliability was compromised because of overfitting and unreliable predictions. To emphasize the interpretability of the developed model and address the data biases surrounding the current lack of diversity in the available demographics, this work closely focused on a specific function: face detection. ML systems should be developed to be visible and interpretable if we want clinicians to build confidence in them. In future work, further study should be done using newer sophisticated and explainable AI methods like deep learning models coupled with interpretable frameworks to enhance earlier CKD diagnosis and clinical acceptability.

UmaRani & Nidhian (2024), Existing research developed a hybrid machine learning framework by using the Whale Optimization Algorithm (WOA) and three classifiers, namely Random Forest Classifier (WOA-RFC), Logistic Regression classifier (WOA-LRC) and Decision Tree Classifier (WOA-DTC) for CKD prediction. The maximum accuracy of 98.8% was achieved by the WOA-RFC model over the hybrid models on the UCI-CKD dataset. These results help us to show that early prediction of CKD diagnosis is improved by having metaheuristic optimization and ensemble learning under WOA-RFC. However, the model's ability to assess clinical data and identify disease-specific patterns shows that the intelligent hybrid system may be a successful source of timelier, more accurate, and more scalable diagnostic tools. Evolutionary algorithms have the potential to be used to fine-tune model parameters for better healthcare results, and this study demonstrates exactly that.

Ghosh et al. (2024), The CKD prediction was compared using XGBoost, Random Forest, Logistic Regression and AdaBoost. The best-performing combination of algorithms is in the form of a hybrid model. It achieved an accuracy of 94.99%, precision of 95.21%, recall of 95.11%, and F1-score of 95.32%, along with an AUROC of 95.56, much higher than that of solo classifiers. This demonstrates that the hybrid model can improve the ability to predict CKD risk and increase the risk assessment's robustness. According to the research, ensemble and hybrid learning may also help identify early CKD and inform clinical decision-making. The Hybrid Model should also be tested on more diverse and larger datasets to ensure generalizability. They suggest adding advanced clinical variables and longitudinal studies to improve chronic illness management and encourage proactive therapies to evaluate the model's performance as a long-term predictor.

Kumar et al. (2024), In another research, K-Nearest Neighbors (KNN), Support Vector Machine (SVM), Artificial Neural Networks (ANN), Random Forest (RF), and XGBoost were compared for CKD prediction. Other models besides Random Forest and XGBoost are outperformed in predicting performance. They were both stable and generalized well to training data of various fractions: Random Forest had 98.2% accuracy, and XGBoost 96.7% for model performance evaluation, accuracy, precision, recall, F1 score and accurate positive/false negative analysis along with ROC curves were used. These findings show that ensemble models can capture complicated data linkages and are an appropriate method for CKD prediction systems. This study demonstrates the need for, and utility of, model selection and validation for clinically useful diagnostic tools.

Sonwalkar & Tamane (2024), In recent research, a comparison of Support Vector Machine (SVM), Decision Tree (DT) and Convolutional Neural Network (CNN) models was made for CKD prediction. Using the Chi-Squared (Chi-2) method, the study improved model accuracy and reliability to manage missing values, encoding and select features. What the CNN model predicted was the most accurate and error-proof method out of all three models assessed; it predicted 119 out of 120 instances. CNN can recognize complicated, non–linear clinical data patterns and, therefore, is a viable method for early diagnosis of CKD. The research did not address the issues associated with a lack of data quality and model generalizability across different patient groups. However, the study did not optimize or compare the model to ensemble approaches that could produce better-predicted outcomes. Because of these limitations, universal diagnostic frameworks cannot be developed without developing more sophisticated or hybrid model validation and testing.

Mazumdar et al. (2025), Adaptive Boosting (ADAB), CatBoost Algorithm (CA), K-Nearest Neighbor (KNN), Probability Boosted Regression (PBR) and Wide-Deep Decision Trees (WADET) were compared in another study for CKD prediction. These models were assessed using accuracy, precision, recall and F1 score on the Kaggle CKD dataset. Among all the conventional and boosting techniques, the Hybrid Optimization Search Model (HOSM) coupled with WADET (HOSM-WADET) presents the highest cumulative accuracy of 98.77%. The results of this study indicate that hybrid optimization can improve CKD prediction. The research addressed none of those implementation issues, model overfitting, repeatability and generalizability across different patient groups. None of the studies were concerned with the long-term applicability of the presented models in the clinical domain, such as across diverse demographic groups with different health profiles and access to treatment. This discrepancy also demonstrates that the HOSM-WADET model has potential and requires further validation and longitudinal research to establish its clinical reliability and potential.

Mandava et al. (2024), A comparison of logistic regression, support vector machine (SVM), random forest, artificial neural network (ANN), and Gaussian naive Bayesian was carried out to predict CKD. The study included twenty-five clinical characteristics related to the diagnosis of CKD. The best-predicted accuracy by the ANN algorithm is 100%, and this ability to understand complex patterns and predict medical outcomes makes this method the best choice. On the other hand, Gaussian Naive Bayes had the lowest accuracy value of 94.0%. Algorithm selection is emphasized, as models differ in data complexity, interpretability or accuracy. The study results make it possible to compare and choose the machine learning models for CKD progression prediction depending on the clinical needs and the data availability for healthcare practitioners.

Ramesh & Kalyanasundaram (2024), Four ensemble tree-based models are used to predict CKD as Random Forest, Extra Trees, AdaBoost & XGBoost, and their performance is compared with KNN, SVM and ANN. The prediction accuracy of the ensemble models was less than that of KNN, SVM, and ANN, with a percentage accuracy of 99.2%. With rigorous preprocessing and efficient feature selection, non-ensemble classifiers can generally classify CKD or non-CKD patients. The research pointed out how these algorithms could automate clinical early-stage CKD identification and risk assessment. The accuracy of these models is perfect over many trials, and they are, therefore, suitable for use in decision support systems to improve nephrology patient outcomes and resource use.

Table 1. Comparative Analysis of ML Algorithms for CKD Prediction

Sr. No	Citation	Methodology	Result Discussion
1	(Rahat et al., 2024; Ghauri et al., 2024)	Logistic Regression	Accuracy: 98.21% - 100%
2	(Gogoi & Valan, 2024)	Decision Trees	Accuracy: 95.83% - 97.50%
3	(Kumar et al., 2024)	Random Forests	Accuracy: 98.2% - 98.46%
4	(Kafle et al., 2025)	XGBoost	Accuracy: 95.78% - 99.17%
5	(Ghosh et al., 2024)	LightGBM	Accuracy: 94.99%
6	(Miah et al., 2023)	AdaBoost	Accuracy: 95%
7	(Bindu et al., 2024)	CatBoost	Accuracy: 97%
8	(Sonwalkar & Tamane, 2024)	CNN	Reported highest correct predictions among DL models
9	(Ramesh & Kalyanasundaram, 2024)	DNN	Reported higher performance than traditional ML models
10	(UmaRani & Nidhian, 2024)	WOA-RF	Accuracy: 98.8%
11	(Mazumdar et al., 2025)	HOSM-WADET	Accuracy: 98.77%
12	(Miah et al., 2023)	Hybrid Model	Accuracy: 99%

Although many achievements have been made in machine learning applications for chronic kidney disease (CKD) prediction, there are still some research gaps. However, most of these studies are limited to small or single-source datasets such as the UCI CKD dataset, which restricts the ability to generalize to different patient populations. Moreover, although reported accuracy can be high, few models include explainable AI techniques, impeding clinical adoption. Despite most models requiring only a binary classification, longitudinal prediction of CKD progression, in particular, has not been explored. Furthermore, the potential hybrid and deep learning-based models are not externally validated on real-world data. Finally, they rarely deploy into CDSS and real healthcare settings, indicating the need for further interpretable, scalable, and clinically applicable CKD prediction frameworks.

4. MACHINE LEARNING ALGORITHMS FOR CDK

Machine learning (ML) algorithms have been widely used to bring a service to healthcare for the early detection and prediction of chronic kidney disease (CKD). These algorithms can find patterns in complex clinical data and pave the way for early and accurate diagnosis. Some of the ML models that we experimented on CKD prediction include traditional classifiers (Logistic Regression, Support Vector Machine (SVM), K-Nearest Neighbor (KNN)), ensemble (Random Forest (RF), AdaBoost, XGBoost). Furthermore, recent approaches have explored some techniques such as Artificial Neural Networks (ANN) and Convolutional Neural Networks (CNN) due to their ability to learn features directly from raw channels automatically. The algorithms come with different strengths in accuracy, interpretability, and scalability. In this part, we give an overview of the most widely used ML algorithms for CKD prediction, and the working principles, strengths, and weaknesses of these algorithms in clinical practice are discussed.

The first step is collecting all the required clinical and laboratory data from different sources (e.g. hospitals, health records, etc.) or picking up CSV datasets from the publicly available datasets (e.g. UCI CKD dataset). The data for this problem typically includes patient demographics, test results (serum creatinine, albumin, hemoglobin, etc.), and diagnosis history. After the data is collected, it enters the Data Preprocessing phase, where it is cleaned and transformed to be quality and usable. In this step, we will deal with missing values, transform categorical features to numerical ones, normalize numerical values (e.g. min-max scaling) and select the most relevant features using techniques like Chi-Squared or feature importance ranking. Again, from data preprocessing, the data is fed into the Model Training phase wherein we introduce machine learning algorithms like Logistic Regression, Random Forest, XGBoost or Artificial Neural Networks trained on a labelled dataset to learn patterns of the presence or progression of CKD. The model is next evaluated on performance metrics such as accuracy, precision, an, and Cando to determine robustness. In the last stage, CKD Prediction, we use the optimized model to predict whether a given new or never-seen patient record has CKD to support early detection and clinical decision-making. This step can be integrated into the clinical decision support system (CDDS) for real-time diagnosis and intervention. In figure 2, show the General Architecture for CDK.

Figure 2. System Flow for CDK

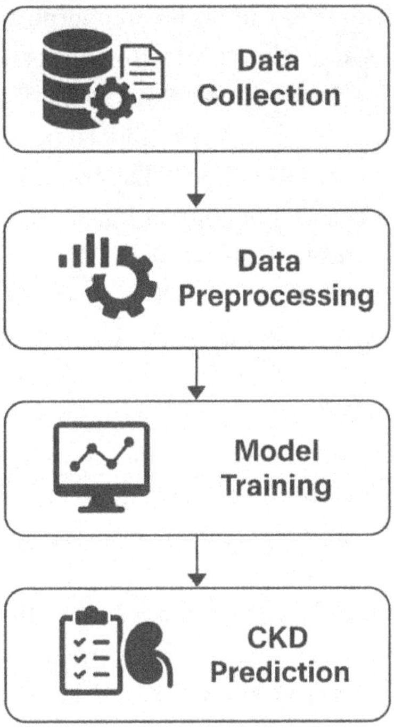

Logistic Regression (LR): The versatile yet straightforward Logistic Regression algorithm can be applied for tasks like CKD prediction since it's a broadly used classification algorithm for medical diagnosis. In this case, it is a binary outcome to model where it models whether or not a patient has CKD based on one or more input features. It uses the logistic (sigmoid) function to map predictions between 0 and 1 as probabilities. LR is often favoured in clinical applications because it is interpretational and easy to implement; in many cases, it is crucial to understand the contribution of each feature (such as age, blood pressure or creatinine level) independently. However, it may be ineffective when the underlying data relationships are not linear.

Support Vector Machine (SVM): A robust supervised learning algorithm, Support Vector Machine, tries to find the best hyperplane that classifies the data points into two different classes. SVM can support CKD prediction, classifying patients as having and without the disease by relying on several clinical factors. It works exceptionally well in high-dimensional spaces and can deal with non-linear data using kernel functions. SVM typically provides high accuracy in CKD classification tasks but can be computationally expensive with large datasets and does not provide the interpretability necessary in some healthcare settings.

Random Forest (RF): Random Forest is an ensemble learning algorithm that, during training, builds multiple decision trees and outputs the class that is the mode of the classes output by the individual trees. Since it can manage missing values, reduce overfitting and deal well with extensive feature sets, it is highly effective for CKD prediction. It also provides feature importance to identify which clinical parameters are the most important to CKD diagnosis. RF has high performance, stability, and ease of use in healthcare applications.

XGBoost (Extreme Gradient Boosting): XGBoost is an advanced Boosting algorithm that, by building the trees sequentially, corrects the previous tree's errors and, hence, is very accurate & efficient. For CKD prediction, iterative optimization of prediction performance is done by minimizing classification errors using XGBoost. It works well with imbalanced datasets, which is usually the case with CKD data. Furthermore, XGBoost also contains techniques used for regularization that prevent the model's overfitting, making it an ideal fit for high-stakes domains such as healthcare. Unfortunately, they are not derivable and are hard to tune and interpret compared to simpler models, such as logistic regression.

K-Nearest Neighbors (KNN): A K-Nearest Neighbors is a non-parametric, instance-based learning algorithm that performs the classification task on a data point by voting among the majority class amongst its 'k' nearest neighbours in the feature space. KNN makes creative on the basis of the patient's clinical parameters by comparing them to clinical parameters of existing labelled data to predict CKD. The system is easy to implement and does not rely on prior data distribution. KNN is, however, prone to noise and irrelevant features and is sensitive to its choice of 'k' and distance metric.

Figure 3. Machin learning algorithms for CDK

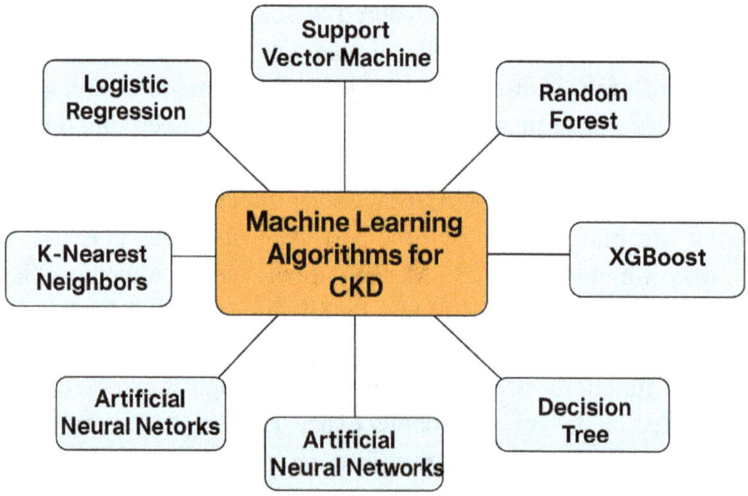

Artificial Neural Networks (ANN): Artificial neural networks are similar to the human brain and have three layers: input, hidden, and output. As such, they can be used for CKD prediction when there are many interrelated clinical features, where they can model complex, non-linear relationships in the data. Backpropagation is used in ANN to learn weights to minimize prediction error. It is especially effective when other methods fail to capture deeper interactions between features fully. ANNS provide high output accuracy at a price of larger data needs and computational power, with their 'black box' nature posing clinical trust limitations unless paired with explainable AI techniques.

Decision Tree (DT): A rule-based algorithm splits the data into branches concerning feature thresholds and ends with classification results. DTs can be used in CKD diagnosis to derive if-then rules from clinic parameters such as serum creatinine, blood pressure, and interpretable hemoglobin levels. Their attractivity in clinical settings is due to their being easy to visualize and understand. However, standalone decision trees tend to overfit and lack generalization ability when there is noisy or imbalanced training data.

5. ACCURACY ANALYSIS OF VARIOUS MACHIN LEARNING ALGORITHMS

The table 2, presents the comparative analysis, which shows the performance of accuracy of ten machine learning algorithms used to predict chronic kidney disease (CKD). The effectiveness of each algorithm was evaluated based on the results that they produced from available literature regarding the ability of each algorithm to detect and classify diseases early. Our results indicate that Artificial Neural Networks achieved the highest accuracy at 100%, demonstrating their ability to model complex non-linear relationships in medical datasets. This implies that ANN might be an appropriate CKD-predicting method when significant and high-quality data are available. K-Nearest Neighbors (KNN) also had an accuracy of 99.2%, while Support Vector Machine (SVM) trailed closely with 99.2% accuracy. This shows (KNN and SVM) to be very strong and robust classifiers and the effectiveness of feature selection and preprocessing techniques used for these classifiers.

An accuracy of 98.2% was achieved by Random Forest, one of the widely used ensembles learning methods which prove to be a reliable and interpretable model for healthcare applications. Also, for the same reason, Logistic Regression, which is transparent and straightforward, achieved an accuracy of 98.33%, which makes it a good candidate to be used in clinical environments where interpretability is essential. Meanwhile, the XGBoost, a strong boosting algorithm, had a slightly lower accuracy of 96.7% but remains on par with the rest as it is regularized and speedy.

The ease of use and visual interpretability of the Decision Tree algorithm made it possible to reach 95.83% accuracy. Still, like any other algorithm, it tends to overfit the dataset with a complex structure. The performance of hybrid models and optimization-enhanced approaches like WOA-RF (98.8%) and HOSM-WADET (98.77%) indicates that machine learning combined with a metaheuristic search algorithm enhances the prediction power of the model. In these cases, the general hybrid model, including the strengths of various classifiers, showed an accuracy of 94.99%. Although slightly lower, it is good and improves with the tuning.

In Figure 4 and 5, the analysis reveals that while advanced deep learning models like ANN show superior accuracy, traditional ML algorithms such as SVM, RF, and LR also offer highly reliable results. Moreover, hybrid optimization techniques show significant promise, emphasizing the potential for combining various methods to enhance predictive performance. These findings are critical for selecting appropriate models based on specific clinical requirements, computational constraints, and the need for interpretability.

Table 2. Accuracy Analysis of Machine Learning Algorithms for CKD

Sr. No	Algorithm	Accuracy (%)
1	Logistic Regression	98.33
2	Support Vector Machine (SVM)	99.2
3	Random Forest	98.2
4	XGBoost	96.7
5	Decision Tree	95.83
6	K-Nearest Neighbors (KNN)	99.2
7	Artificial Neural Networks (ANN)	100.0
8	Whale Optimization Algorithm + RF (WOA-RF)	98.8
9	Hybrid Optimization Search Model (HOSM-WADET)	98.77
10	Hybrid Model	94.99

Figure 4. Line Chart-Accuracy Comparison of ML Algorithms for CKD

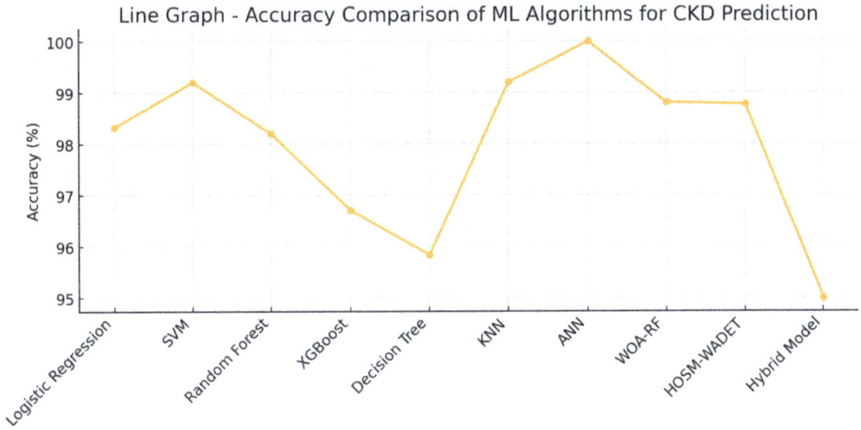

Figure 5. Bar Chart-Accuracy Analysis of Machine Learning Algorithms for CKD

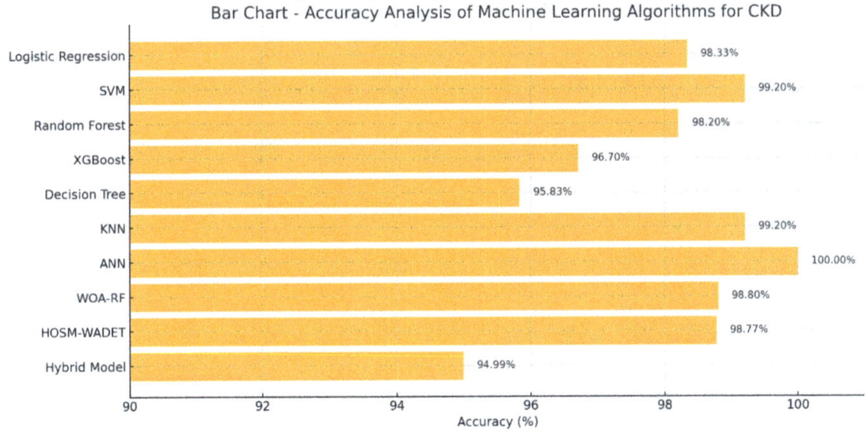

6. CONCLUSION

In this chapter, we have provided comprehensive views of the machine learning techniques that can be applied for predicting and early predicting chronic kidney disease (CKD). In the first part, CKD and its progressive nature were described at the beginning. Also stressed was the importance of early detection for reducing CKD morbidity and mortality. The part that explained the stages of CKD was how

REFERENCES

Bindu, H., Valluru, D., Vachhani, H., Kumar, M. S., Ganesh, D., & Neelima, P. (2024).. . *Comparison of Novel Machine Learning Algorithms for Predicting Chronic Renal Disease., 1–5.* Advance online publication. DOI: 10.1109/iccigst60741.2024.10717629

Ghauri, A. R. K., Danish, M., Nadeem, L., Amin, Y., Mahmood, T., Sheraz, M., Chuah, T. C., & Roslee, M. (2024). Detection of Chronic Kidney Disease Using Machine Learning. 1–6. https://doi.org/DOI: 10.1109/mecon62796.2024.10776391

Ghosh, B. P., Imam, T., Anjum, N., Mia, M. T., Siddiqua, C. U., Sharif, K. S., & Hossain, M. Z. (2024). Advancing chronic kidney disease prediction: Comparative analysis of machine learning algorithms and a hybrid model. *Journal of Computer Science and Technology Studies*, *6*(3), 15–21.

Gogoi, P., & Valan, J. A. (2024). Interpretable Machine Learning for Chronic Kidney Disease Prediction: A SHAP and Genetic Algorithm-Based Approach. *Biomedical Materials & Devices*, •••, 1–19.

Kafle, S., Sah, R. S., Smriti, K. C., & Khadka, S. R. (2025). Leveraging Machine Learning Algorithms for Prediction Chronic Kidney Disease: A Comparative Analysis. *J Clin Res Case Stud*, *3*(1), 1–8.

Kumar, R. R., Mudepalli, S., Sujay, V., Lande, J., & Mohmmad, S. (2024, June). An Empirical Method For Chronic Kidney Disease Prediction. In *2024 15th International Conference on Computing Communication and Networking Technologies (ICCCNT)* (pp. 1-5). IEEE.

Mandava, S., Vinta, S. R., Ghosh, H., & Rahat, I. S. (2024). A comparative analysis of machine learning and deep learning approaches for prediction of chronic kidney disease progression. *EAI Endorsed Trans Internet Things*, *10*, 11.

Mazumdar, H., Khondakar, K. R., Das, S., Halder, A., & Kaushik, A. (2025). Artificial intelligence for personalized nanomedicine; from material selection to patient outcomes. *Expert Opinion on Drug Delivery*, *22*(1), 85–108. PMID: 39645588

Miah, J., Rahat, Md. A. R., Ahmed, A. H., Shahriyar, M. A., & Lipu, E. R. (2023). A Comparative Analysis of Machine Learning Approaches for Chronic Kidney Disease Detection. 1–6. https://doi.org/DOI: 10.1109/iceeie59078.2023.10334765

Rahat, M. A. R., Islam, M. T., Cao, D. M., Tayaba, M., Ghosh, B. P., Ayon, E. H., & Bhuiyan, M. S. (2024). Comparing machine learning techniques for detecting chronic kidney disease in early stage. *Journal of Computer Science and Technology Studies*, *6*(1), 20–32.

Ramesh, S. M., & Kalyanasundaram, P. (2024, July). A Machine Learning Perspective for Predicting Chronic Kidney Disease. In *2024 2nd International Conference on* Sustainable Computing and Smart Systems (ICSCSS) (pp. 989-993). IEEE.

Sonwalkar, M. S., & Tamane, S. C. (2024, June). Comparison of Machine Learning Models for Chronic Kidney Disease Prediction using UCI dataset. In *2023 4th International Conference on Intelligent Technologies (CONIT)* (pp. 1-6). IEEE.

UmaRani. V., & Nidhian, T. (2024). A Hybrid Whale Optimisation Algorithm and Machine Learning Technique for Chronic Kidney Disease Prediction. In *Multidisciplinary Approaches for Sustainable Development* (pp. 59-63). CRC Press.

Compilation of References

Abascal, J., Lazkano, E., & Sierra, B. (2005). Behavior-based indoor navigation. Ambient Intelligence for Scientific Discovery: Foundations, Theories, and Systems, 263-285.

Abbas, A., Abdelsamea, M. M., & Gaber, M. M. (2021). Classification of COVID-19 in chest X-ray images using DeTraC deep convolutional neural network. *Applied Intelligence*, *51*(1), 854–864. DOI: 10.1007/s10489-020-01829-7 PMID: 34764548

Ahmed, N., & Sabir, M. (2015). A superior achievement of brain tumor detection using segmentation based on F-transform. In *2015 IEEE International Conference*. IEEE.

Akhtar, M. N., Iqbal, M. K., & Abid, M. S. (2025). Renal vision advanced kidney disease detection using attention-powered ensemble CNNs. Physical Education. *Health and Social Sciences*, *3*(1), 31–42.

Akter, S., Habib, A., Islam, M. A., Hossen, M. S., Fahim, W. A., Sarkar, P. R., & Ahmed, M. (2021). Comprehensive performance assessment of deep learning models in early prediction and risk identification of chronic kidney disease. *IEEE Access : Practical Innovations, Open Solutions*, *9*, 165184–165206. DOI: 10.1109/ACCESS.2021.3134130

Alalawi, H. H., & Alsuwat, M. S. (2021). Detection of cardiovascular disease using machine learning classification models. *International Journal of Engineering Research & Technology (Ahmedabad)*, *10*(7), 151–157.

Al-Galal, S. A. Y., Alshaikhli, I. F. T., & Abdulrazzaq, M. M. (2021). MRI brain tumor medical images analysis using deep learning techniques: A systematic review. *Health and Technology*, *11*(2), 267–282. DOI: 10.1007/s12553-020-00514-6

Alikhan, J. S., Alageswaran, R., & Miruna Joe Amali, S. (2023). Self-attention convolutional neural network optimized with season optimization algorithm espoused chronic kidney diseases diagnosis in big data system. *Biomedical Signal Processing and Control*, *85*, 105011. Advance online publication. DOI: 10.1016/j.bspc.2023.105011

Ali, M., Gilani, S. O., Waris, A., Zafar, K., & Jamil, M. (2020). Brain tumour image segmentation using deep networks. *IEEE Access : Practical Innovations, Open Solutions*, *8*, 153589–153598. DOI: 10.1109/ACCESS.2020.3018160

Almustafa, K. M. (2021). Prediction of chronic kidney disease using different classification algorithms. *Informatics in Medicine Unlocked*, *24*, 100631. Advance online publication. DOI: 10.1016/j.imu.2021.100631

Amini, P., Ramezanali, F., Parchehbaf-Kashani, M., Maroufizadeh, S., Omani-Samani, R., & Ghaheri, A. (2021). Factors associated with in vitro fertilization live birth outcome: A comparison of different classification methods. *International Journal of Fertility & Sterility*, *15*(2), 128. PMID: 33687166

Antonelo, E. A., & Schrauwen, B. (2014). On learning navigation behaviors for small mobile robots with reservoir computing architectures. *IEEE Transactions on Neural Networks and Learning Systems*, *26*(4), 763–780. PMID: 25794381

Antony, L., Azam, S., Ignatious, E., Quadir, R., Beeravolu, A. R., Jonkman, M., & De Boer, F. (2021). A comprehensive unsupervised framework for chronic kidney disease prediction. *IEEE Access : Practical Innovations, Open Solutions*, *9*, 126481–126501. DOI: 10.1109/ACCESS.2021.3109168

Aprilianto, D. (2020). SVM optimization with correlation feature selection based binary particle swarm optimization for diagnosis of chronic kidney disease. *Journal of Soft Computing Exploration*, *1*(1), 24–31.

Ashley, E. A. (2016). Towards precision medicine. *Nature Reviews. Genetics*, *17*(9), 507–522. PMID: 27528417

Asif, S., Wenhui, Y., Jin, H., & Jinhai, S. (2020). Classification of COVID-19 from chest X-ray images using deep convolutional neural network. In 2020 IEEE 6th International Conference on Computer and Communications (ICCC) (pp. 426–433). IEEE. https://doi.org/DOI: 10.1109/ICCC51575.2020.9344870

Ayadi, W., Elhamzi, W., Charfi, I., & Atri, M. (2021). Deep CNN for brain tumor classification. *Neural Processing Letters*, *53*(1), 671–700. DOI: 10.1007/s11063-020-10398-2

Bachelder, I. A., & Waxman, A. M. (1995). A view-based neurocomputational system for relational map-making and navigation in visual environments. *Robotics and Autonomous Systems, 16*(2-4), 267–289.

Baghdadi, N. A., Farghaly Abdelaliem, S. M., Malki, A., Gad, I., Ewis, A., & Atlam, E.-S. (2023). Advanced machine learning techniques for cardiovascular disease early detection and diagnosis. *Journal of Big Data, 10*(1), 144. Advance online publication. DOI: 10.1186/s40537-023-00814-8

Bai, Q., Su, C., Tang, W., & Li, Y. (2022). Machine learning to predict end stage kidney disease in chronic kidney disease. *Scientific Reports, 12*(1), 8377. Advance online publication. DOI: 10.1038/s41598-022-11757-6 PMID: 35589908

Bajaj, D., Kumari, R., & Bansal, P. (2023). Risk level prediction for maternal health using machine learning algorithms. In *2023 International Conference on Communication, Security and Artificial Intelligence (ICCSAI)* (pp. 405-409). IEEE.

Bashshur, R. L., Shannon, G. W., & Smith, B. R.. (2014). The empirical foundations of telemedicine interventions in primary care. *Telemedicine Journal and e-Health, 20*(5), 342–375. PMID: 27128779

Baur, K., Schättin, A., de Bruin, E. D., Riener, R., Duarte, J. E., & Wolf, P. (2018). Trends in robot-assisted and virtual reality-assisted neuromuscular therapy: A systematic review of health-related multiplayer games. *Journal of Neuroengineering and Rehabilitation, 15*, 1–19. PMID: 30454009

Bhak, Y., Lee, Y. H., Kim, J., Lee, K., Lee, D., Jang, E. C., & Jang, E. (2025). Diagnosis of chronic kidney disease using retinal imaging and urine dipstick data: Multimodal deep learning approach. *JMIR Medical Informatics, 13*(1), e55825. PMID: 39924305

Bideau, B., Kulpa, R., Vignais, N., Brault, S., Multon, F., & Craig, C. (2009). Using virtual reality to analyze sports performance. *IEEE Computer Graphics and Applications, 30*(2), 14–21. PMID: 20650707

Bindu, H., Valluru, D., Vachhani, H., Kumar, M. S., Ganesh, D., & Neelima, P. (2024).. . *Comparison of Novel Machine Learning Algorithms for Predicting Chronic Renal Disease., 1–5*. Advance online publication. DOI: 10.1109/iccigst60741.2024.10717629

Bodenheimer, T., & Sinsky, C. (2014). From triple to quadruple aim: Care of the patient requires care of the provider. *Annals of Family Medicine, 12*(6), 573–576. PMID: 25384822

Burra, L. R., Tumuluru, P., Bonam, J., Raju, S. H., Nalajala, S., & Borra, S. P. R. (2025). Innovative application of conditional deep convolutional generative adversarial networks to enhance chronic kidney disease diagnosis with uneven datasets. In Smart factories for Industry 5.0 transformation (pp. 71–87).

Chandra, S. K., & Bajpai, M. K. (2018). Effective algorithm for benign brain tumor detection using fractional calculus. In Proceedings of TENCON 2018 - 2018 IEEE Region 10 Conference. IEEE.

Chandralekha, E., Vinodhini, S., Kandasamy, V., Rama, P., Ravikumar, S., & Saravanan, T. R. (2023). An extensive machine learning framework employing ensemble classifiers for heart disease detection. In 2023 3rd International Conference on Innovative Mechanisms for Industry Applications (ICIMIA) (pp. 973–978). IEEE. https://doi.org/DOI: 10.1109/ICIMIA60397.2023.10084912

Chang, Y.-J., Lin, C.-H., & Chien, Y.-C. (2025). Predicting the risk of chronic kidney disease based on uric acid concentration in stones using biosensors integrated with a deep learning-based ANN system. *Talanta*, *283*, 127077. PMID: 39476796

Chiang, W., & Jin, Y. (2011, January). Toward a meta-model of behavioral interaction for designing complex adaptive systems. In *International Design Engineering Technical Conferences and Computers and Information in Engineering Conference* (Vol. 54792, pp. 1077-1088).

Cojocaru, A. M., Bucea-Manea- oni , R., Jianu, A., Dumangiu, M. A., Alexandrescu, L. U., & Cojocaru, M. (2022). The role of physical education and sports in modern society supported by IoT—A student perspective. *Sustainability*, *14*(9), 5624.

Collins, F. S., & Varmus, H. (2015). A new initiative on precision medicine. *The New England Journal of Medicine*, *372*(9), 793–795. PMID: 25635347

Crider, K. S., Qi, Y. P., & Yeung, L. F.. (2022). Folic acid and the prevention of birth defects: 30 years of opportunity and controversies. *Annual Review of Nutrition*, *42*, 423–452. PMID: 35995050

Cui, X., Chen, N., Zhao, C., Li, J., Zheng, X., Liu, C., Yang, J., Li, X., Yu, C., Liu, J., & Liu, X. (2023). An adaptive weighted attention-enhanced deep convolutional neural network for classification of MRI images of Parkinson's disease. *Journal of Neuroscience Methods*, *394*, 109884. Advance online publication. DOI: 10.1016/j.jneumeth.2023.109884 PMID: 37207799

Dasare, A., & S, H. (2021). Covid19 infection detection and classification using CNN on chest X-ray images. In 2021 IEEE International Conference on Distributed Computing, VLSI, Electrical Circuits and Robotics (DISCOVER) (pp. 292–296). IEEE. https://doi.org/DOI: 10.1109/DISCOVER52564.2021.9663614

de Moura, E. P. (2021). SARS-CoV-2 CT-scan dataset. Kaggle. https://www.kaggle.com/datasets/plameneduardo/sarscov2-ctscan-dataset

Debal, D. A., & Sitote, T. M. (2022). Chronic kidney disease prediction using machine learning techniques. *Journal of Big Data*, *9*(1), 109. Advance online publication. DOI: 10.1186/s40537-022-00657-5

Dhanve, V., & Kumar, M. (2017). Detection of brain tumor using k-means segmentation based on object labeling algorithm. In *2017 IEEE International Conference on Power, Control, Signals and Instrumentation Engineering (ICPCSI)*. IEEE.

Diamanti, A., Papadakis, S., & Schoretsaniti, S.. (2019). Smoking cessation in pregnancy: An update for maternity care practitioners. *Tobacco Induced Diseases*, *17*, 57. PMID: 31582946

Esteva, A., Kuprel, B., & Novoa, R. A.. (2017). Dermatologist-level classification of skin cancer with deep neural networks. *Nature*, *542*(7639), 115–118. PMID: 28117445

Evripidou, S., Georgiou, K., Doitsidis, L., Amanatiadis, A. A., Zinonos, Z., & Chatzichristofis, S. A. (2020). Educational robotics: Platforms, competitions and expected learning outcomes. *IEEE Access : Practical Innovations, Open Solutions*, *8*, 219534–219562.

Ezhilarasi, R., & Varalakshmi, P. (2018). Tumor detection in the brain using faster R-CNN. In 2018 2nd International Conference on I-SMAC (IoT in Social, Mobile, Analytics and Cloud) (I-SMAC) (pp. 388–392). IEEE. https://doi.org/DOI: 10.1109/I-SMAC.2018.8653736

Ferguson, T., Ravani, P., Sood, M. M., Clarke, A., Komenda, P., Rigatto, C., & Tangri, N. (2022). Development and external validation of a machine learning model for progression of CKD. *Kidney International Reports*, *7*(8), 1772–1781. DOI: 10.1016/j.ekir.2022.05.028 PMID: 35967110

Fernandez-Leon, J. A., Acosta, G. G., & Rozenfeld, A. (2014). How simple autonomous decisions evolve into robust behaviours?: A review from neurorobotics, cognitive, self-organized and artificial immune systems fields. *Bio Systems*, *124*, 7–20. PMID: 25149273

Geng, T.-T., Chen, J.-X., Lu, Q., Wang, P.-L., Xia, P.-F., Zhu, K., & Li, Y. (2024). Nuclear magnetic resonance–based metabolomics and risk of CKD. *American Journal of Kidney Diseases*, *83*(1), 9–17. DOI: 10.1053/j.ajkd.2023.06.007 PMID: 37678743

Georgakopoulou, V. E., & Diamanti, A. (2024). Artificial intelligence for smoking cessation in pregnancy. *Cureus*, *16*(7). PMID: 39100043

George, C., Echouffo-Tcheugui, J. B., Jaar, B. G., Okpechi, I. G., & Kengne, A. P. (2022). The need for screening, early diagnosis, and prediction of chronic kidney disease in people with diabetes in low- and middle-income countries—A review of the current literature. *BMC Medicine*, *20*(1), 247. Advance online publication. DOI: 10.1186/s12916-022-02466-5 PMID: 35915501

Ghauri, A. R. K., Danish, M., Nadeem, L., Amin, Y., Mahmood, T., Sheraz, M., Chuah, T. C., & Roslee, M. (2024). Detection of Chronic Kidney Disease Using Machine Learning. 1–6. https://doi.org/DOI: 10.1109/mecon62796.2024.10776391

Ghosh, B. P., Imam, T., Anjum, N., Mia, M. T., Siddiqua, C. U., Sharif, K. S., & Hossain, M. Z. (2024). Advancing chronic kidney disease prediction: Comparative analysis of machine learning algorithms and a hybrid model. *Journal of Computer Science and Technology Studies*, *6*(3), 15–21.

Glatstein, I., Chavez-Badiola, A., & Curchoe, C. L. (2023). New frontiers in embryo selection. *Journal of Assisted Reproduction and Genetics*, *40*(2), 223–234. PMID: 36609943

Gobhinath, S., Anandkumar, S., Dhayalan, R., Ezhilbharathi, P., & Haridharan, R. (2021). Human brain tumor detection and classification by medical image processing. In 2021 7th International Conference on Advanced Computing and Communication Systems (ICACCS). IEEE. https://doi.org/DOI: 10.1109/ICACCS51430.2021.9441877

Gogoi, P., & Valan, J. A. (2024). Interpretable Machine Learning for Chronic Kidney Disease Prediction: A SHAP and Genetic Algorithm-Based Approach. *Biomedical Materials & Devices*, •••, 1–19.

Gomes, R., Carmo, T., Braga, K., Santos, A., Andrade, C., & Andrade, E. (2024). Arduino programming of an educational robotic platform applied in radiological accident simulation. *Brazilian Journal of Radiation Sciences*, *12*(1), e2395–e2395.

Gururaj, H. L., Flammini, F., Srividhya, S., Chayadevi, M. L., & Selvam, S. (Eds.). (2024). Computer science engineering: *Proceedings of the 1st International Conference on Computing and Intelligent Information Systems (ICCIIS 2024)*, Bangalore, India, 19–20 April, 2024 (Vol. 2). CRC Press. https://doi.org/DOI: 10.1201/9781003565024

He, D. Q., Wang, H. B., & Li, P. F. (2018, May). Robot path planning using improved rapidly-exploring random tree algorithm. In 2018 IEEE Industrial Cyber-Physical Systems (ICPS) (pp. 181-186). IEEE.

Hebli, A., & Gupta, S. (2017). Brain tumor prediction and classification using support vector machine. In *2017 IEEE International Conference on Advances in Computing, Communications and Informatics (ICACCI)*. IEEE.

Heidari, M., Mirniaharikandehei, S., Khuzani, A. Z., Danala, G., Qiu, Y., & Zheng, B. (2020). Improving the performance of CNN to predict the likelihood of COVID-19 using chest X-ray images with preprocessing algorithms. *International Journal of Medical Informatics*, *144*, 104284. Advance online publication. DOI: 10.1016/j.ijmedinf.2020.104284 PMID: 32992136

Hood, L., & Friend, S. H. (2011). Predictive, personalized, preventive, participatory (P4) cancer medicine. *Nature Reviews. Clinical Oncology*, *8*(3), 184–187. PMID: 21364692

Hussain, E., Hasan, M., Rahman, M. A., Lee, I., Tamanna, T., & Parvez, M. Z. (2021). CoroDet: A deep learning based classification for COVID-19 detection using chest X-ray images. *Chaos, Solitons, and Fractals*, *142*, 110495. Advance online publication. DOI: 10.1016/j.chaos.2020.110495 PMID: 33250589

Ibrahim, D. M., Elshennawy, N. M., & Sarhan, A. M. (2021). Deep-chest: Multi-classification deep learning model for diagnosing COVID-19, pneumonia, and lung cancer chest diseases. *Computers in Biology and Medicine*, *132*, 104348. Advance online publication. DOI: 10.1016/j.compbiomed.2021.104348 PMID: 33774272

Iftikhar, H., Khan, M., Khan, Z., Khan, F., Alshanbari, H. M., & Ahmad, Z. (2023). A comparative analysis of machine learning models: A case study in predicting chronic kidney disease. *Sustainability*, *15*(3), 2754. Advance online publication. DOI: 10.3390/su15032754

Iliyas, I. I., Isa, A., Zarma, M. L., & Dauda, B. A. (2025). Deep learning in predicting genetic disorders: A case study of diabetic kidney disease. In *Deep learning in genetics and genomics* (pp. 329–347). Academic Press.

Illingworth, P. J., Venetis, C., Gardner, D. K., Nelson, S. M., Berntsen, J., Larman, M. G., & Hardarson, T. (2024). Deep learning versus manual morphology-based embryo selection in IVF: A randomized, double-masked noninferiority trial. *Nature Medicine*, •••, 1–7. PMID: 39122964

Iqbal, S., Qureshi, A. N., Alhussein, M., Aurangzeb, K., Zubair, M., & Hussain, A. (2025). A novel reciprocal domain adaptation neural network for enhanced diagnosis of chronic kidney disease. *Expert Systems: International Journal of Knowledge Engineering and Neural Networks*, *42*(2), e13825.

Islam, M. A., Majumder, M. Z. H., & Hussein, M. A. (2023). Chronic kidney disease prediction based on machine learning algorithms. *Journal of Pathology Informatics*, *14*, 100189. Advance online publication. DOI: 10.1016/j.jpi.2023.100189 PMID: 36714452

Ismail, W. N. (2023). Snake-efficient feature selection-based framework for precise early detection of chronic kidney disease. *Diagnostics (Basel)*, *13*(15), 2501. Advance online publication. DOI: 10.3390/diagnostics13152501 PMID: 37568865

Jabbar, F. A., & Rithanya, K. S. (2021). Risks of chronic kidney disease prediction using various data mining algorithms. International Journal of Informatics [INJIIS-COM]. *Information System and Computer Engineering*, *2*(2), 165–177.

Jacquline, M. L., & Sudha, N. (2024). Chronic kidney disease classification using entropy based butterfly optimization and improved artificial neural network algorithm: Preprocessing, feature selection, clustering, and disease prediction. *Journal of Angiotherapy*, *8*(6), 1–12.

Jerlin Rubini, L., & Perumal, E. (2020). Efficient classification of chronic kidney disease by using multi-kernel support vector machine and fruit fly optimization algorithm. *International Journal of Imaging Systems and Technology*, *30*(3), 660–673. DOI: 10.1002/ima.22406

Jerlin Rubini, L., & Perumal, E. (2022). Oppositional firefly optimization based optimal feature selection in chronic kidney disease classification using deep neural network. *Journal of Ambient Intelligence and Humanized Computing*, *13*(4), 1799–1810. DOI: 10.1007/s12652-020-02824-5

Jia, G., Lam, H.-K., & Xu, Y. (2021). Classification of COVID-19 chest X-ray and CT images using a type of dynamic CNN modification method. *Computers in Biology and Medicine*, *134*, 104425. Advance online publication. DOI: 10.1016/j.compbiomed.2021.104425 PMID: 33971427

Joo, S. H., Manzoor, S., Rocha, Y. G., Bae, S. H., Lee, K. H., Kuc, T. Y., & Kim, M. (2020). Autonomous navigation framework for intelligent robots based on a semantic environment modeling. *Applied Sciences (Basel, Switzerland)*, *10*(9), 3219.

Kabir, M. A. (2020). Early-stage brain tumor detection on MRI image using a hybrid technique. In 2020 IEEE Region 10 Symposium (TENSYMP). IEEE.

Kafle, S., Sah, R. S., Smriti, K. C., & Khadka, S. R. (2025). Leveraging Machine Learning Algorithms for Prediction Chronic Kidney Disease: A Comparative Analysis. *J Clin Res Case Stud*, *3*(1), 1–8.

Kaur, N., & Sharma, M. (2017). Brain tumor detection using self-adaptive K-means clustering. In *2017 International Conference on Energy, Communication, Data Analytics and Soft Computing (ICECDS)*. IEEE.

Keesara, S., Jonas, A., & Schulman, K. (2020). Covid-19 and health care's digital revolution. *The New England Journal of Medicine*, *382*(23), e82. PMID: 32240581

Khalid, H., Khan, A., Khan, M. Z., Mehmood, G., & Qureshi, M. S. (2023). Machine learning hybrid model for the prediction of chronic kidney disease. *Computational Intelligence and Neuroscience*, *2023*, 9266889. Advance online publication. DOI: 10.1155/2023/9266889 PMID: 36959840

Kitagawa, Y., Ishikura, T., Song, W., Mae, Y., Minami, M., & Tanaka, K. (2009, August). Human-like patient robot with chaotic emotion for injection training. In 2009 ICCAS-SICE (pp. 4635-4640). IEEE.

Kohane, I. S. (2015). Ten things we have to do to achieve precision medicine. *Science Translational Medicine*, *7*(316), 316cm316. Advance online publication. DOI: 10.1126/scitranslmed.aab1328 PMID: 26138968

Kovacs, P. (2014). Embryo selection: The role of time-lapse monitoring. *Reproductive Biology and Endocrinology*, *12*, 1–11. PMID: 25510244

Kumar, A. (2024). IoT-Enhanced Spy Robotics Bridging Security Gaps. In Shaping the Future of Automation With Cloud-Enhanced Robotics (pp. 343-358). IGI Global.

Kumar, R. R., Mudepalli, S., Sujay, V., Lande, J., & Mohmmad, S. (2024, June). An Empirical Method For Chronic Kidney Disease Prediction. In *2024 15th International Conference on Computing Communication and Networking Technologies (ICCCNT)* (pp. 1-5). IEEE.

Kumari, S., & Singh, S. K. (2022). An ensemble learning-based model for effective chronic kidney disease prediction. In *2022 International Conference on Computing, Communication, and Intelligent Systems (ICCCIS)* (pp. 162–168). IEEE. https://doi.org/DOI: 10.1109/ICCCIS56430.2022.10037562

Kumar, S., Dhir, R., & Chaurasia, N. (2021). Brain tumor detection analysis using CNN: A review. In *2021 International Conference on Artificial Intelligence and Smart Systems (ICAIS)* (pp. 1061–1067). IEEE. https://doi.org/DOI: 10.1109/ICAIS50930.2021.9395920

Lakshmi, K. L., Umadevi, M., & Bellamkonda, L. P. (2025). Optimized truncated singular value decomposition and hybrid deep neural network with random forest for automated disease prediction. *Biomedical Signal Processing and Control*, *100*, 107010.

Lau, H. Y., & Wong, V. W. (2007). An immunity approach to strategic behavioral control. *Engineering Applications of Artificial Intelligence*, *20*(3), 289–306.

Lipschuetz, M., Guedalia, J., Cohen, S. M., Unger, R., Yagel, S., & Sompolinsky, Y. (2024). Machine learning in electronic health records: Identifying high-risk obstetric patients pre and during labor. In *Innovation in Applied Nursing Informatics* (pp. 3–7). IOS Press.

Ma, J., Wang, J., Lu, L., Sun, Y., Feng, M., Shen, P., Jiang, Z., Hong, S., & Zhang, L. (2025). Development and validation of a dynamic kidney failure prediction model based on deep learning: A real-world study with external validation. arXiv preprint arXiv:2501.16388.

Mandava, S., Vinta, S. R., Ghosh, H., & Rahat, I. S. (2024). A comparative analysis of machine learning and deep learning approaches for prediction of chronic kidney disease progression. *EAI Endorsed Trans Internet Things*, *10*, 11.

Mandula, A., & Vijaya Kumar, B. S. (2024). Integrated feature selection and ensemble learning for heart disease detection: A 2-tier approach with ALAN and ET-ABDF machine learning model. *International Journal of Information Technology : an Official Journal of Bharati Vidyapeeth's Institute of Computer Applications and Management*, *16*(7), 4489–4503. DOI: 10.1007/s41870-024-02245-6

Mark, R. S. (2020). The impact of artificial intelligence on patient monitoring. *IEEE Transactions on Biomedical Engineering*, *67*(5), 1234–1245. DOI: 10.1109/TBME.2019.2942998

Mateus, N., Abade, E., Coutinho, D., Gómez, M. Á., Peñas, C. L., & Sampaio, J. (2024). Empowering the Sports Scientist with Artificial Intelligence in Training, Performance, and Health Management. *Sensors (Basel), 25*(1), 139. PMID: 39796930

Mazumdar, H., Khondakar, K. R., Das, S., Halder, A., & Kaushik, A. (2025). Artificial intelligence for personalized nanomedicine; from material selection to patient outcomes. *Expert Opinion on Drug Delivery, 22*(1), 85–108. PMID: 39645588

Mehta, V., Batra, N., Goyal, S., Kaur, A., Dudekula, K. V., & Victor, G. J. (2024). Machine Learning based Exploratory Data Analysis (EDA) and Diagnosis of Chronic Kidney Disease (CKD). *EAI Endorsed Transactions on Pervasive Health and Technology, 10*(1), e4.

Miah, J., Rahat, Md. A. R., Ahmed, A. H., Shahriyar, M. A., & Lipu, E. R. (2023). A Comparative Analysis of Machine Learning Approaches for Chronic Kidney Disease Detection. 1–6. https://doi.org/DOI: 10.1109/iceeie59078.2023.10334765

Miao, Z., & Ge, G. (2023). Research on the Development of Sports in the Age of Artificial Intelligence. power, 5(7), 6-11.

Miotto, R., Wang, F., Wang, S., Jiang, X., & Dudley, J. T. (2018). Deep learning for healthcare: Review, opportunities, and challenges. *Briefings in Bioinformatics, 19*(6), 1236–1246. PMID: 28481991

Mittal, P., Sharma, Y. K., Lilhore, U. K., Simaiya, S., Saleem, K., & Ghith, E. S. (2025). Advanced Hybrid Machine Learning Model for Accurate Detection of Cardiovascular Disease. *International Journal of Computational Intelligence Systems, 18*(1), 1–20.

Mittelstadt, B. D., Allo, P., Taddeo, M., Wachter, S., & Floridi, L. (2016). The ethics of algorithms: Mapping the debate. *Big Data & Society, 3*(2), 2053951716679679.

Montag, M., Toth, B., & Strowitzki, T. (2013). New approaches to embryo selection. *Reproductive Biomedicine Online, 27*(5), 539–546. PMID: 23933036

Morley, J., Machado, C. C., Burr, C., Cowls, J., Joshi, I., Taddeo, M., & Floridi, L. (2020). The ethics of AI in health care: A mapping review. *Social Science & Medicine, 260*, 113172. PMID: 32702587

Na, Y. K., & Oh, S. Y. (2003). Hybrid control for autonomous mobile robot navigation using neural network based behavior modules and environment classification. *Autonomous Robots, 15*, 193–206.

Obermeyer, Z., & Emanuel, E. J. (2016). Predicting the future—Big data, machine learning, and clinical medicine. *The New England Journal of Medicine*, *375*(13), 1216–1219. DOI: 10.1056/NEJMp1606181 PMID: 27682033

Pal, S. (2023). Chronic kidney disease prediction using machine learning techniques. *Biomedical Materials & Devices*, *1*, 534–540. DOI: 10.1007/s44174-022-00027-y

Panda, P. K., & Sharma, R. (2024). Transforming maternal healthcare: Harnessing the power of artificial intelligence for improved outcomes and access. *World Journal of Advanced Research and Reviews*, *23*(1), 662–666.

Parveen, G., Joshi, P., Uniyal, Y., & Rawat, S. (2024). Contribution of artificial intelligence to improving women's health in pregnancy. In *Artificial Intelligence and Machine Learning for Women's Health Issues* (pp. 121–135). Academic Press.

Patel, D. J., Chaudhari, K., Acharya, N., Shrivastava, D., & Muneeba, S. (2024). Artificial intelligence in obstetrics and gynecology: Transforming care and outcomes. *Cureus*, *16*(7), e64725. PMID: 39156405

Pavan Kumar, V. S., Yadla, J., Parvatham, N. K., Lokesh Kumar, P., Tulluri, U., & Amrutha, K. (2025). Optimized predictive modelling for chronic kidney disease: A hybrid ensemble approach with bacterial foraging optimization and SMOTE. In 2025 6th International Conference on Mobile Computing and Sustainable Informatics (ICMCSI) (pp. 988–994). IEEE.

Pavitha, N., Dardige, R., Patil, V., Pawar, A., & Shah, B. (2023, December). Obstacle Detection Using Arduino Board and Bluetooth Control. In International Conference on Information and Communication Technology for Competitive Strategies (pp. 297-307). Singapore: Springer Nature Singapore.

Pereira Mendes, C., & Lim, N. T. L. (2024). EcoLiDAR: An economical LiDAR scanner for ecological research. *PLoS One*, *19*(6), e0298712. PMID: 38917132

Pitkin, R. M. (2007). Folate and neural tube defects. *The American Journal of Clinical Nutrition*, *85*, 285S–288S. PMID: 17209211

Polydoros, A. S., & Nalpantidis, L. (2017). Survey of model-based reinforcement learning: Applications on robotics. *Journal of Intelligent & Robotic Systems*, *86*(2), 153–173.

Pradeepa, P., & Jeyakumar, M. K. (2024). Chronic kidney disease prediction using improved deep belief network with local search nearest neighbour optimization. *Computer Methods in Biomechanics and Biomedical Engineering. Imaging & Visualization*, *11*(7), 2292085. Advance online publication. DOI: 10.1080/21681163.2024.2292085

Praveen, S. P., Jyothi, V. E., Anuradha, C., Venugopal, K., Shariff, V., & Sindhura, S. (2024). Chronic kidney disease prediction using ML-based Neuro-Fuzzy model. *International Journal of Image and Graphics*, *24*(6), 2340013. Advance online publication. DOI: 10.1142/S021946782340013X

Puri, A., Mathur, R., & Nayar, K. D. (2024). AI-powered fertility assessment tool. *International Journal of Science and Research Archive*, *12*(1), 742–744.

Qiu, J., Li, P., Dong, M., Xin, X., & Tan, J. (2019). Personalized prediction of live birth before the first in vitro fertilization treatment: A machine learning method. *Journal of Translational Medicine*, *17*, 1–8. PMID: 31547822

Rahat, M. A. R., Islam, M. T., Cao, D. M., Tayaba, M., Ghosh, B. P., Ayon, E. H., & Bhuiyan, M. S. (2024). Comparing machine learning techniques for detecting chronic kidney disease in early stage. *Journal of Computer Science and Technology Studies*, *6*(1), 20–32.

Rahman, M. A. (2020). Artificial intelligence in healthcare: A comprehensive review. *IEEE Access : Practical Innovations, Open Solutions*, *8*, 12345–12360. DOI: 10.1109/ACCESS.2020.2969709

Rahman, M. L., Reza, A. W., & Shabuj, S. I. (2022). An internet of things-based automatic brain tumor detection system. *Indonesian Journal of Electrical Engineering and Computer Science*, *25*(1), 214–222. DOI: 10.11591/ijeecs.v25.i1.pp214-222

Raihen, M. N., & Akter, S. (2024). Comparative assessment of several effective machine learning classification methods for maternal health risk. *Computational Journal of Mathematical and Statistical Sciences*, *3*(1), 161–176.

Raikwar, S., Fehrmann, J., & Herlitzius, T. (2022). Navigation and control development for a four-wheel-steered mobile orchard robot using model-based design. *Computers and Electronics in Agriculture*, *202*, 107410.

Rajkomar, A., Dean, J., & Kohane, I. (2019). Machine learning in medicine. *The New England Journal of Medicine*, *380*(14), 1347–1358. PMID: 30943338

Raj, T., Hanim Hashim, F., Baseri Huddin, A., Ibrahim, M. F., & Hussain, A. (2020). A survey on LiDAR scanning mechanisms. *Electronics (Basel)*, *9*(5), 741.

Ramesh, S. M., & Kalyanasundaram, P. (2024, July). A Machine Learning Perspective for Predicting Chronic Kidney Disease. In *2024 2nd International Conference on* Sustainable Computing and Smart Systems (ICSCSS) (pp. 989-993). IEEE.

Ramspek, C. L., Evans, M., Wanner, C., Drechsler, C., Chesnaye, N. C., Szymczak, M., & Krajewska, M.EQUAL Study Investigators. (2021). Kidney failure prediction models: A comprehensive external validation study in patients with advanced CKD. *Journal of the American Society of Nephrology*, *32*(5), 1174–1186. DOI: 10.1681/ASN.2020071077 PMID: 33685974

Ramu, K., Patthi, S., Prajapati, Y. N., Ramesh, J. V. N., Banerjee, S., Brahma Rao, K. B. V., & Alzahrani, S. I. (2025). Hybrid CNN-SVM model for enhanced early detection of chronic kidney disease. *Biomedical Signal Processing and Control*, *100*, 107084. Advance online publication. DOI: 10.1016/j.bspc.2024.107084

Rashed-Al-Mahfuz, M., Haque, A., Azad, A., Alyami, S. A., Quinn, J. M. W., & Moni, M. A. (2021). Clinically applicable machine learning approaches to identify attributes of chronic kidney disease (CKD) for use in low-cost diagnostic screening. *IEEE Journal of Translational Engineering in Health and Medicine*, *9*, 1–11. DOI: 10.1109/JTEHM.2021.3073629 PMID: 33948393

Rath, A., Mishra, D., & Panda, G. (2021). LSTM-based cardiovascular disease detection using ECG signal. In Cognitive informatics and soft computing: Proceedings of CISC 2020 (pp. 133–142). Springer Singapore. https://doi.org/DOI: 10.1007/978-981-16-1056-1_12

Robot, M. (2024). Discourse analysis and communication strategy of sport learning: a systematic review assisted with VOSviewer. Retos: nuevas tendencias en educación física, deporte y recreación, (61), 430-439.

Rubini, L. J., & Perumal, E. (2020). Hybrid kernel support vector machine classifier and grey wolf optimization algorithm based intelligent classification algorithm for chronic kidney disease. *Journal of Medical Imaging and Health Informatics*, *10*(10), 2297–2307. DOI: 10.1166/jmihi.2020.3192

Saadati, S. A. (2023). Recent innovations in sports physiology: Shaping the future of athletic performance. *Health Nexus*, *1*(2), 15–27.

Salih, M., Austin, C., Warty, R. R., Tiktin, C., Rolnik, D. L., Momeni, M., & Horta, F. (2023). Embryo selection through artificial intelligence versus embryologists: A systematic review. *Human Reproduction Open*, *2023*(3), hoad031. PMID: 37588797

Sara, S. B. V. J., & Kalaiselvi, K. (2019). Ant colony optimization (ACO) based feature selection and extreme learning machine (ELM) for chronic kidney disease detection. *International Journal of Advanced Studies of Scientific Research*, *4*(1).

Sawhney, R., Malik, A., Sharma, S., & Narayan, V. (2023). A comparative assessment of artificial intelligence models used for early prediction and evaluation of chronic kidney disease. *Decision Analytics Journal, 6*, 100169. Advance online publication. DOI: 10.1016/j.dajour.2023.100169

Sezer, V., & Gokasan, M. (2012). A novel obstacle avoidance algorithm:"Follow the Gap Method". *Robotics and Autonomous Systems*, *60*(9), 1123–1134.

Sheridan, T. B. (2016). Human–robot interaction: Status and challenges. *Human Factors*, *58*(4), 525–532. PMID: 27098262

Shifa, H. A., Mojumdar, M. U., Rahman, M. M., Chakraborty, N. R., & Gupta, V. (2024). Machine learning models for maternal health risk prediction based on clinical data. In *2024 11th International Conference on Computing for Sustainable Global Development (INDIACom)* (pp. 1312-1318). IEEE.

Shorewala, V. (2021). Early detection of coronary heart disease using ensemble techniques. *Informatics in Medicine Unlocked*, *26*, 100655. Advance online publication. DOI: 10.1016/j.imu.2021.100655

Singh, K. (2021). Evolution of patient monitoring systems: From traditional to AI-driven. *Journal of Healthcare Engineering*, *11*(2), 123–135. DOI: 10.1155/2021/8899123

Sitaraman, S. R., Alagarsundaram, P., Gattupalli, K., Gollavilli, V. S. B. H., Nagarajan, H., & Ajao, L. A. (2024). Advanced IoMT-enabled chronic kidney disease prediction leveraging robotic automation with autoencoder-LSTM and fuzzy cognitive maps. *International Journal of Modern Electronics and Communication Engineering*, *12*(3), 1–20.

Sonwalkar, M. S., & Tamane, S. C. (2024, June). Comparison of Machine Learning Models for Chronic Kidney Disease Prediction using UCI dataset. In *2023 4th International Conference on Intelligent Technologies (CONIT)* (pp. 1-6). IEEE.

Subasi, A., Alickovic, E., & Kevric, J. (2017). Diagnosis of chronic kidney disease by using random forest. In CMBEBIH 2017: Proceedings of the International Conference on Medical and Biological Engineering 2017 (pp. 589–594). Springer Singapore. https://doi.org/DOI: 10.1007/978-981-10-4166-2_89

Sufian, M. A., Hamzi, W., Hamzi, B., Sagar, A. S., Rahman, M., Varadarajan, J., Hanumanthu, M., & Azad, M. A. K. (2024). Innovative machine learning strategies for early detection and prevention of pregnancy loss: The vitamin D connection and gestational health. *Diagnostics (Basel)*, *14*(9), 920. PMID: 38732334

Swami, M., & Verma, D. (2020). An algorithmic detection of brain tumor using image filtering and segmentation of various radiographs. In 2020 7th International Conference on Signal Processing and Integrated Networks (SPIN). IEEE.

Swathikrishna, M. R., Sriram, S., & Subha, B. (2023). Pre-eclampsia risk prediction using machine learning algorithms. In *International Conference on Information and Communication Technology for Competitive Strategies* (pp. 71-80). Singapore: Springer Nature Singapore.

Tani, J. (1996). Model-based learning for mobile robot navigation from the dynamical systems perspective. *IEEE Transactions on Systems, Man, and Cybernetics. Part B, Cybernetics*, *26*(3), 421–436. PMID: 18263044

Terrada, O., Hamida, S., Cherradi, B., Raihani, A., & Bouattane, O. (2020). Supervised machine learning based medical diagnosis support system for prediction of patients with heart disease. *Advances in Science, Technology and Engineering Systems Journal*, *5*(5), 269–277. DOI: 10.25046/aj050534

Thakkar, D., Gandhi, V. C., & Trivedi, D. (2024). Forecasting maternal women's health risks using random forest classifier. In *2024 International Conference on Inventive Computation Technologies (ICICT)* (pp. 961-965). IEEE.

Theilgaard Lassen, J., Fly Kragh, M., Rimestad, J., Nygård Johansen, M., & Berntsen, J. (2023). Development and validation of deep learning-based embryo selection across multiple transfer days. *Scientific Reports*, *13*(1), 4235. PMID: 36918648

Tian, T., Kong, F., Yang, R., Long, X., Chen, L., Li, M., & Qiao, J. (2023). A Bayesian network model for predicting low or failed fertilization in assisted reproductive technology based on extensive clinical real-world data. *Reproductive Biology and Endocrinology*, *21*(1), 8. PMID: 36703171

Tiwari, R. G., Agarwal, A. K., & Jain, V. (2023). Leveraging machine learning for comprehensive analysis of maternal health: Predicting health risks and improving antenatal care. In *International Conference on Mobile Radio Communications & 5G Networks* (pp. 287-297). Singapore: Springer Nature Singapore.

Togunwa, T. O., Babatunde, A. O., & Abdullah, K. (2023). Deep hybrid model for maternal health risk classification in pregnancy: Synergy of ANN and random forest. *Frontiers in Artificial Intelligence*, *6*, 1213436. PMID: 37476504

Topol, E. J. (2019). High-performance medicine: The convergence of human and artificial intelligence. *Nature Medicine*, *25*(1), 44–56. DOI: 10.1038/s41591-018-0300-7 PMID: 30617339

Ukrit, M. F., Jeyavathana, R. B., Rani, A. L., & Chandana, V. (2024). Maternal health risk prediction with machine learning methods. In *2024 Second International Conference on Emerging Trends in Information Technology and Engineering (ICE-TITE)* (pp. 1-9). IEEE.

Umans, E., Dewilde, K., Williams, H., Deprest, J., & Van den Bosch, T. (2024). Artificial intelligence in imaging in the first trimester of pregnancy: A systematic review. *Fetal Diagnosis and Therapy*, *51*(4), 343–356. PMID: 38493764

UmaRani. V., & Nidhian, T. (2024). A Hybrid Whale Optimisation Algorithm and Machine Learning Technique for Chronic Kidney Disease Prediction. In *Multidisciplinary Approaches for Sustainable Development* (pp. 59-63). CRC Press.

Vaishnavee, K. B., & Amshakala, K. (2015). An automated MRI brain image segmentation and tumor detection using SOM-clustering and proximal support vector machine classifier. In *2015 IEEE International Conference on Engineering and Technology (ICETECH)*. IEEE.

Van Slobbe, R., Herrmannova, D., Boeke, D. J., Lima-Walton, E. S., Abu-Hanna, A., & Vagliano, I. (2025). Multimodal convolutional neural networks for the prediction of acute kidney injury in the intensive care. *International Journal of Medical Informatics*, •••, 105815. PMID: 39914070

Vatavu, A., Rahm, M., Govindachar, S., Krehl, G., Mantha, A., Bhavsar, S. R., & Maile, M. (2020). From particles to self-localizing tracklets: A multilayer particle filter-based estimation for dynamic grid maps. *IEEE Intelligent Transportation Systems Magazine*, *12*(4), 149–168.

Vayena, E., Blasimme, A., & Cohen, I. G. (2018). Machine learning in medicine: Addressing ethical challenges. *PLoS Medicine*, *15*(11), e1002689. DOI: 10.1371/journal.pmed.1002689 PMID: 30399149

Vogiatzi, P., Pouliakis, A., & Siristatidis, C. (2019). An artificial neural network for the prediction of assisted reproduction outcome. *Journal of Assisted Reproduction and Genetics*, *36*, 1441–1448. PMID: 31218565

Webster, J. G. (2009). *Medical instrumentation: Application and design* (4th ed.). Wiley.

Wen, J. Y., Liu, C. F., Chung, M. T., & Tsai, Y. C. (2022). Artificial intelligence model to predict pregnancy and multiple pregnancy risk following in vitro fertilization-embryo transfer (IVF-ET). *Taiwanese Journal of Obstetrics & Gynecology*, *61*(5), 837–846. PMID: 36088053

Xi, Q., Yang, Q., Wang, M., Huang, B., Zhang, B., Li, Z., & Jin, L. (2021). Individualized embryo selection strategy developed by stacking machine learning model for better in vitro fertilization outcomes: An application study. *Reproductive Biology and Endocrinology*, *19*, 1–10. PMID: 33820565

Yang, T., & Song, J. (2018). An automatic brain tumor image segmentation method based on the U-net. In 2018 IEEE 4th International Conference on Computer and Communications (ICCC) (pp. 1600–1604). IEEE.

Yang, H., Liu, F., Ma, Y., & Di, M. (2022). Clinical pregnancy outcomes prediction in vitro fertilization women based on random forest prediction model: A nested case-control study. *Medicine*, *101*(49), e32232. PMID: 36626443

Yang, M., Sun, X., Jia, F., Rushworth, A., Dong, X., Zhang, S., & Liu, B. (2022). Sensors and sensor fusion methodologies for indoor odometry: A review. *Polymers*, *14*(10), 2019. PMID: 35631899

Yaonan, W., Yimin, Y., Xiaofang, Y., Yi, Z., Yuanli, Z., Feng, Y., & Lei, T. (2011). Autonomous mobile robot navigation system designed in dynamic environment based on transferable belief model. *Measurement*, *44*(8), 1389–1405.

Yaseen, I., & Rather, R. A. (2024). A theoretical exploration of artificial intelligence's impact on feto-maternal health from conception to delivery. *International Journal of Women's Health*, •••, 903–915. PMID: 38800118

Yewale, D., Vijayaragavan, S. P., & Bairagi, V. K. (2023). An effective heart disease prediction framework based on ensemble techniques in machine learning. *International Journal of Advanced Computer Science and Applications*, *14*(2), 1–10.

Zhou, R., & Wu, F. (2023). Inheritance and Innovation Development of Sports based on Deep Learning and Artificial Intelligence. *IEEE Access : Practical Innovations, Open Solutions*, *11*, 116511–116523.

About the Contributors

Dattatray Takale is Assistant Professor, Department of Computer Engineering at Vishwakarma Institute of Information Technology, Pune, India. Dr. Dattatray G. Takale obtained his Ph.D. in computer science and engineering. He has 10 + years of teaching and research experience. His research interests include Machine Learning, Data science, Wireless sensor Network, Natural lang. processing, data warehousing, mining, computer networks, and network security. He is currently employed by VIIT Pune, as an Assistant Professor. His has more than 6 years of teaching experience and 3 years industry experience. He has 21 patents, 20+ research publications, and authored/edited 4+ books with Springer, CRC Press, local and international publisher.

Parikshit Mahalle is a senior member IEEE and is Professor, Head of Department of Artificial Intelligence and Data Science at Vishwakarma Institute of Information Technology, Pune, India. He completed his Ph. D from Aalborg University, Denmark and continued as Post Doc Researcher at CMI, Copenhagen, Denmark. He has 23 + years of teaching and research experience. He is a member of the Board of Studies in Computer Engineering, Ex-Chairman Information Technology, Savitribai Phule Pune University and various Universities and autonomous colleges across India. He has 12 patents, 200+ research publications (Google Scholar citations-2500 plus, H index-23 and Scopus Citations are 1300 plus with H index -16, Web of Science H index - 10) and authored/edited 50+ books with Springer, CRC Press, Cambridge University Press, etc. He is editor in chief for IGI Global –International Journal of Rough Sets and Data Analysis, Inter-science International Journal of Grid and Utility Computing, member-Editorial Review Board for IGI Global – International Journal of Ambient Computing and Intelligence and reviewer for various journals and conferences of the repute. His research interests are Machine Learning, Data Science, Algorithms, Internet of Things, Identity Management and Security. He is guiding 8 PhD students in the area of IoT and machine learning and recently, FIVE students have successfully defended their PhD under his supervision. He is also the recipient of "Best Faculty Award" by Sinhgad Institutes and Cognizant Technologies Solutions. He has delivered 200 plus lectures at national and international level.

Bipin Sule is a Management & Education strategist, held various academic & administrative positions in his educational career of 28+ years, currently working as Chief Executive Officer (CEO) of a well-known educational Group – Vishwakarma Institutes & University – Pune Maharashtra India, heading the operations of - 5 campus, 15+ Institutes, approx. 2500+ staff & 25,000+ students from many states of India and more than 35+ countries offering more than 60+ courses.

Vivek S. Deshpande holds Bachelors and Masters of Engineering in Electronics & Telecommunications from Pune University and Doctorate from Nagpur University, India. He Has got 31 years of experience comprises of Industry and academia as well. Currently Dr. Vivek is Director at Vishwakarma Institute of Information Technology, VIIT, Pune. He worked in VIT, Pune as Professor and Head for Computer Engineering Department. He is doing his research in Wireless Sensor Networks, embedded systems, IoT, Industry 4.0, High-Performance Computer Networks and AI Machine learning as well. Dr Vivek is pursued his Post-Doctoral Research Fellowship from Technical University of Sofia, Bulgaria, Europe. He published more than 70 papers in international journals and conferences of repute. He filed 24 Indian patents, and all are published now. Dr Vivek is working on many research projects which tackles more social and industrial problems. Vivek is Senior member of IEEE, Pune Section (R10, India). He chairs Education Society and Industry Relations for Pune Chapter. He is also a Chair of conference committee of Pune Chapter. Dr Vivek recently developed a Wireless Network Lab in Pune. This lab is now converted into Centre of Excellence for IoT. There are three verticals namely e-Health, Precision Agriculture and Smart City are targeted in this COE. Dr Vivek is also active member of the IP Lab, where industry automation is collaborated with Artificial intelligence and machine learning technology. Their expertise in High Performance Computer Network, Real Time Embedded Systems, Distributed Systems, Mathematical foundation for IT, Research and Data Analytics, Wireless Communication Technologies, Wireless Sensor Networks, 5G IoT, Industry 4.0, Technology Management, Block Chain Technology will be invaluable to the project's success.

Nilesh P. Sable is a senior member IEEE and working as Associate Professor, Head Department of Computer Science & Engineering (Artificial Intelligence) at Vishwakarma Institute of Information Technology, Pune, India. He has completed his Ph.D. in Computer Science & Engineering on Research Problem Statement

"Study on Relationship Standard Mining Calculations in Data Mining" in 2018. He has 16 + years of teaching and research experience. He is guiding 4 Ph.D. students in the area of Machine Learning, Federated Learning and IoT under his supervision from Savitribai Phule Pune University, Pune. He is working as Research Advisory Committee (RAC) Member for various Research Centres. He is a reviewer for various journals and conferences of the repute. His research interests are Data Mining, Image Processing, Machine Learning, Cognitive Computing, Internet of Things, Networking and Security. He has published 100+ papers in National, International conferences and Journals. He had Filed and Published 21 Patents and 18 Copyrights. He has authored books published by National/International publishers. He is also the recipient of the "Distinguished Performance Award" by Vishwakarma Institute of Information Technology. He has delivered 75+ lectures at national and international level.

***

Sanket Anbhule is having Computer science background and passionate about exploring things Deep Learning and Environment Science

Anushka Bhagwat is a B.Tech student of Vishwakarma Institute of Information technology, Pune and her interest lies in Machine Learning and Deep learning

Sushil Bhardwaj is an IT professional with more than 21 years of experience in academics and research. His Educational Qualification is Ph.D (CSE), MCA, M.Tech (ECE), B.E.(ECE) and currently working as Professor at RIMT University, Mandi Gobindgarh (India). His current area of research and interest includes modeling and performance evaluation of computer networks, machine learning, cloud computing, computer architecture, and IoT. He has authored 45 books. He has published more than 32 research papers in various International Journal, National / International Conferences having indexed with SCI, Scopus, ACM etc.

Adarsh Dawkhare is having Computer science background and passionate about exploring things in Machine Learning and Deep Learning

Chitra Joshi is a B.Tech student of Vishwakarma Institute of Information technology, Pune and her interest lies in Machine Learning and Deep learning

Shilpa Kalantri is an accomplished and student focused professor with rich experience of 25 years. She motivates students to pursue academics sincerely and become successful Engineers. She has taught various subjects across Computer Engineering during her teaching career.

Abhishek Kumar is a qualified educator with a Ph.D. (Electronics and Electrical Engineering) completed from Lovely Professional University, M.Tech from VJTI, the University of Mumbai on the qualifying GATE examination, and graduated from Institution of Engineers(India). I am currently associated as an Associate Professor at the VLSI Domain, School of Electrical and Electronics Engineering, Lovely Professional University, India has more than 12 years of teaching and research experience. I have authored more than 25 peer reviewed research articles indexed in SCI, Scopus indexed journals and 12 proceeding in index conferences proceedings. There are 4 book with IEEE/Wiley-SP and authored 8-book chapter. There are 4 copyrights and published 11 patents. I am an Active Reviewer and an Editorial Member of numerous prominent SCI and Scopus indexed journals.

Atharva Pardeshi is a B.Tech student of Vishwakarma Institute of Information technology, Pune and his interest lies in developing the web applications and Machine Learning

Snehal Rathi is an accomplished and student-focused professor with 21 years teaching experience in diverse classroom environments. She inspires students to pursue academic and personal excellence for becoming life-long learners. She has wide experience in the areas of curriculum development and evaluation methodologies. She is awarded Ph.D. in (Computer Engineering) from Vishwakarma University, Pune, India. She is presently working as an associate professor in Computer Engineering department at Vishwakarma Institute of Technology, Pune. She has taught multiple subjects which includes Data Structures, Data Mining and Machine Learning. Her research interest includes machine learning, deep learning, soft computing and human computer interaction.

Pratik Rathod is having Computer science background and passionate about exploring things in ML, Deep Learning and Quantum Computing

Harpreet Singh Bedi, PhD, is an Associate Professor at Lovely Professional University (LPU), Phagwāra, India. He has 15 years of experience in both teaching and industry, specializing in areas such as Communication & Signal Processing, Information and Communication Technology, Cellular Communication, Satellite Communication, Photovoltaic Systems, and Algorithms. His contributions to research and innovation include over 30 published patents, 2 granted patents, and 2 registered copyrights under his name. He has also authored a book and published more than 50 research papers in renowned scientific and technical journals, showcasing his dedication to advancing knowledge in his field.

Index

A

B

C

D

E

F

H

I

M

N

P

R

S

T

W

X

www.ingramcontent.com/pod-product-compliance
Lightning Source LLC
LaVergne TN
LVHW080855300926
849162LV00003B/421